THE CARE ASSISTANT'S GUIDE

to working with

ELDERLY MENTALLY INFIRM PEOPLE

THE CARE ASSISTANT'S GUIDE
to working with
ELDERLY MENTALLY INFIRM PEOPLE

Edited by
Sue Benson
and
Patrick Carr

A Care Concern Publication

First published in 1991 by
Hawker Publications Ltd
13 Park House
140 Battersea Park Road
London SW11 4NB

Reprinted 1992

British Library Cataloguing in Publication Data

A catalogue record for this book is available
from the British Library

ISBN 0-9514649-6-5

Designed by
Richard Souper

Phototypeset by
Just Words Ltd, Brighton

Printed and bound in Great Britain by
Butler and Tanner, Frome, Somerset

*Illustrations in chapters 10 and 15 are redrawn from Keeping the Elderly Moving in Old People's
Homes by Helen Ransome, published by the Centre for Policy on Ageing, and How to Save a Life by
Alan Maryon Davies and Jenny Rogers, published by BBC Books.*

Other titles in this series:
Handbook for Care Assistants – A Practical Guide to Caring for Elderly People
Second Edition (revised) 1992. ISBN 0-9514649-7-3
A Practical Guide to Working with People with Learning Disabilities – A Handbook for
Care Assistants and Support Workers. 1992. ISBN 1-874790-00-0

Contents

Contributors

June Andrews MA RMN RGN is Assistant Director, Policy and Research at the Royal College of Nursing. For most of her clinical nursing career she has been a nurse caring for elderly people in many settings.

Richard Banks BEd (Education and Applied Social Studies) is Programme Head for Social Care at the Central Council for Education and Training in Social Work.

Sue Benson BA RGN gained an honours degree in English at Hull University and qualified as a State Registered Nurse at St George's Hospital, London. She has been involved with Care Concern for seven years as Editor, Consultant and Features Editor, and was previously Deputy Editor of Nursing Mirror. She also works on the nurses' bank at Atkinson Morley's Hospital, Wimbledon.

Theresa Briscoe is a trained nurse who has been working with elderly and elderly mentally ill people for 10 years. She founded the Royal College of Nursing Special Interest Group for Activities Nurses, and won the "Nurse of the Year" award in 1988 for services to nursing elderly people.

Karen Bryan PhD BSc(Hons) MCSLT is a lecturer in acquired communication disorders at the National Hospitals College of Speech Sciences. She previously worked as a speech therapist with elderly people.

Patrick Carr BA PhD RMN SRN RNT is Chief Executive of the Registered Nursing Home Association and former Head of Nursing Studies at Manchester Polytechnic. He has carried out extensive research in the field of psychiatric nursing, served as an elected member of the English National Board (1983-1988) and is president of the Community Psychiatric Nurses Association. He and his wife (both nurses) have run their own nursing home in Cheshire since 1979.

Pauline Crawford RGN, Certificate of the Royal Marsden Hospital, is a general manager for Ashbourne Homes plc. She is also a member of the Royal College of Nursing Executive Committee for care of elderly people.

Stuart J Darby RGN RMN RHV DPSN is Practice Development Nurse within the directorate of community health, Bloomsbury and Islington Health Authority. He has worked as a clinical nurse specialist in mental health and as a health visitor with older people. He is current chair of the Royal College of Nursing membership group, FOCUS: on older people, nursing and mental health.

Steve Goodwin is Clinical Coordinator at Southport Nursing Development Unit. He has previously worked in social sciences, and with elderly people in the voluntary and private sectors and NHS. He directs the award-winning Cosmic Nursing Projects.

Ian Hicken RMN RGN CPNCert worked for several years as a community psychiatric nurse. His work included liaison and consultation with statutory and non-statutory elderly care institutions. He now works as Project Officer HIV/AIDS, Education and Training, for the English National Board for Nursing, Midwifery and Health Visiting.

Alan Higson RMN RCNT CertEd(FE) is Training Manager for Health Care Assistants with Tunbridge Wells Health Authority, and is currently a Control and Restraint Instructor for the South East Thames Regional Health Authority. He has worked with disturbed clients since 1976 and was the first chairman of the Royal College of Nursing's forum for nurses working in secure environments.

Brenda Hooper MA is Manager of Libury Hall residential care home. She was previously a training adviser at the Centre for Policy on Ageing, and is author of *Home Ground*, a handbook on staff training.

Michael Maltby BSc DipClinPsych AFBPS CPsychol is a clinical psychologist with Tunbridge Wells Health Authority. He specialises in work with older people and carers, including staff training and consultancy.

Ruth Manley RGN RCNT worked for many years in the NHS and later with the Royal College of Nursing. She currently acts as an independent nurse adviser on health care projects for older people.

Jane Maxim PhD MA DipCST MCSLT is a senior lecturer at at The National Hospitals College of Speech Sciences. She is a speech therapist whose research area is language change in dementia, and she runs a group for elderly stroke patients.

Teresa Mearing-Smith BSc MB BCh DCH MRCGP is Clinical Assistant in Geriatrics and Dermatology at St Peter's Hospital, Chertsey. She previously worked as a general practitioner, with a special interest in care of older people.

Gwyn Roberts DMS is General Manager for Tadworth Grove nursing and residential home, part of the Court Cavendish Group. She has been involved with elderly confused people for five years, and previously worked in the field of training and information science.

Peter Watkins RMN DN RNT DipHumPsych is a nurse tutor at the Suffolk and Great Yarmouth College of Nursing and Midwifery in Ipswich. He has a wide experience of nursing practice, teaching and counselling and a particular involvement in designing and facilitating personal and interpersonal effectiveness programmes for care staff.

Deirdre Wynne-Harley is Deputy Director of the Centre for Policy on Ageing and is involved in a wide range of consultancies with statutory, voluntary and private sector agencies. Her special interests in the field of older age are design and lifestyle, risk taking and advocacy.

Foreword

by Nori Graham, Consultant in Old Age Psychiatry, The Royal Free Hospital, London, and National Chairman of The Alzheimer's Disease Society

The problem of old age and illness in old age has grown into a crisis in the UK. The number of people over the age of 80 will, it is estimated, increase by half as much again by the year 2000, and this is the group which is most at risk in terms of physical and mental illness. The majority of elderly people live at home, but an increasing proportion of them live on their own. These are the people who are most likely to need residential care if they become ill, especially if they become mentally ill.

Mental disorders can be more crippling than physical illness. An elderly man living on his own who is alert but has severe arthritis or a broken leg can be helped in his home by brief daily visits, but a man who has no memory and no sense of time or place is impossible to help except with 24-hour care.

The two most common mental disorders are depression and dementia. Approximately one in 10 people over the age of 80 is depressed and one in five has a dementia. This means that every one of us probably knows at least one person within the family or neighbourhood with one of these disorders.

Research has shown that in residential units the average age is 85 years. Around two thirds of the residents are suffering from dementia and one half are depressed. Depression and dementia are associated with much greater rates of dependency and problem behaviours such as incontinence, wandering and aggression. It is important that these conditions are identified and diagnosed. Depression is eminently treatable, very common and often overlooked, and the cause of unnecessary suffering. Dementia, on the other hand, is not treatable but an early diagnosis will allow the development of a personalised management plan with advice and support, both for the person suffering and those doing the caring.

Care staff in residential and nursing units need access to courses and training material which will inform them in as practical way as possible about these common mental illnesses, which are now part and parcel of normal care activity. Staff will want to learn how to recognise these disorders, when to refer for an opinion or assessment, and most especially what they themselves can do to help. In particular the behavioural problems associated with these disorders can so often be alleviated if carers understand what is causing them. It is not helpful to see severe memory loss or depression as part of normal ageing. Behavioural problems usually have an understandable cause in the form of a mental illness or underlying physical illness.

The majority of old people are neither depressed nor suffering from dementia. However, caring for those who are demands factual information and understanding; for this reason I welcome the initiative by *Care Concern* to publish this book.

The book seems to me to give a very comprehensive and full account of the problems likely to be faced by care assistants. Readers will absorb a number of important messages. First, every chapter emphasises the individuality of the elderly person. Everyone has their life story, likes and dislikes, and older people are no exception.

Then there is much stress on the quality of the environment and the way that this should allow for individual privacy and personal space. The chapter on diversional activities will be an inspiration to those who like myself often find it difficult to be creative about ways of occupying elderly people at risk of inactivity and boredom. Finally, the contributors do not let the reader forget that elderly people have relatives who have an important role to play after care has become residential.

The contents of this book will make a real difference to the morale and confidence of staff who read it, for they will find much in it to inform and encourage them in their work.

Nori Graham

Introduction

One of the best ways to absorb up-to-date, practice-based knowledge and skills is to attend a study day or seminar taught by working experts in the field. The popularity of *Care Concern's* seminar series for care home staff, Caring for Elderly Mentally Infirm People, initiated by our publisher Richard Hawkins, has proved the success of this approach.

This book is a seminar in print, for all care assistants and health support workers in whatever residential or nursing environment. Every author is an expert with current hands-on experience of caring for confused elderly people in a residential setting. Every author addresses you, the reader, as if you were a learner in their study group. Every author keeps constantly in mind the difficulties and frustrations, as well as the satisfactions, of the work you do from day to day.

Just as at a study day, different personalities with different styles illuminate and reinforce a central consistent approach, so underlying each chapter's detail is one central theme: treat your elderly mentally infirm residents as far as possible as if they were normal. A simple, sound principle of care; not so simple, however, to put into practice. It needs translation into everyday practical guidance for all the caring situations you are likely to meet in your work - the guidance you will find in the pages of this book.

The job titles of care assistant and nursing auxiliary are no longer enough to cover all who do this work. With the advent of National Vocational Qualifications, job titles are in a state of flux. We feel "care assistant" is still the most widely understood term; most authors have adopted this title, intending it to cover those who work in both care homes and hospitals. Similarly we have retained each author's description of the people in their care. Whether "resident", "patient" or "client" is used, it is intended to cover older people in all residential settings.

We are immensely proud of the chapters contained in these pages. The authors' commitment to the goal we all share - better, more informed care for elderly mentally infirm people - shines through the practical detail of their advice. Their enthusiasm and patience has matched the depth of their working knowledge and teaching skill.

We would also like to thank Paulette Prendergast for her committed secretarial assistance, and Sue's husband Christopher for his careful reading and constructive comments on the text.

Sue Benson and Patrick Carr

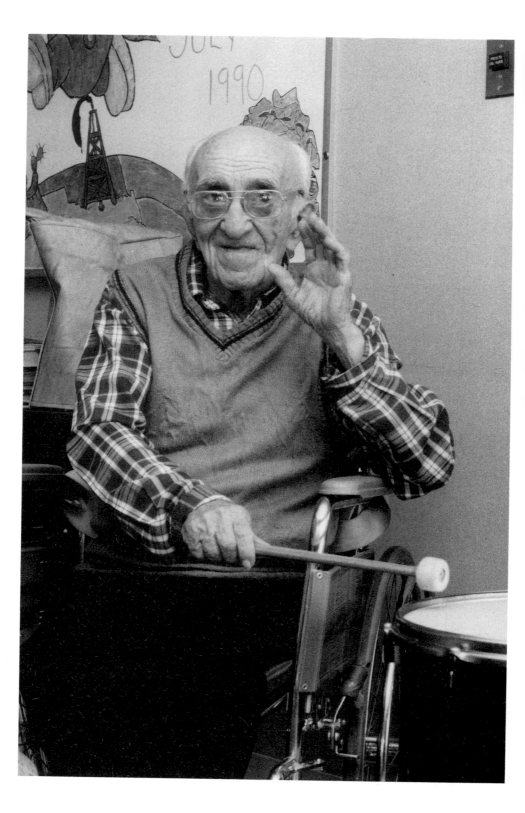

CHAPTER 1

Mental health in older age

by Patrick Carr

The physical, social and psychological changes that old age brings • Mental illness defined • Double trouble with physical and mental problems • When care in a home becomes the best solution

There are two different and quite distinct processes involved in becoming an elderly mentally ill person.

There is, first of all, the fact of being elderly, of growing old. Ageing is of course a natural process, through which we shall all travel if we live long enough.

Old age is not, then, a disease or an illness. It should be considered, in the sense of Shakespeare's "Seven Ages of Man", as just another developmental phase in the life span.

Each one of life's "ages", whether adolescence or the "midlife crisis", has its own problems; this is true of old age as of any other age group. One of the particular problems of growing old is that you have passed through all the other age groups, encountering each age group's set of problems on the way, and that is bound to have left its mark.

Ask yourself the question: who is elderly? I would not mind betting you will answer, "Someone who is quite a bit older than me"! If you were to pose the question to someone quite a bit younger than yourself, they might well think that you are old;

your pictures of "old age" might be quite different.

I think we are agreed, then, that "elderly" or "older" is a relative rather than an absolute concept, and that it would be safe to say that, like beauty, it is in the eye of the beholder.

Age changes

This particular phase of life, however you define it in a relative way, is marked by certain characteristics, and may include the following:

Physical changes

• fading hearing and vision

• loss of teeth

• weakening sense of taste and smell

• decline in muscle and motor strength

• osteoarthritic changes in bones and joints

• connective tissue changes

• wrinkling of skin

• changes in the function of internal organs that may lead to problems like: heart disease, high blood pressure (hypertension), diabetes.

Social and psychological changes

- impairment of memory
- intellectual deterioration
- changed self-image leading to
  - reclusiveness
  - rigid adherence to old ways
  - rejection of new ideas
  - melancholy/depression
  - suspiciousness
  - hostility
- increasing dependence, financial, physical and psychosocial, leading to a loss of self-esteem and creating a basis for possible hostility to and conflict with those nearest and dearest.

You need to bear in mind that the process of growing old will be a process unique to every individual. Each person will age in their own particular way, and at their own particular rate. Writers talk of "the young old" and "the old old", and it is quite clear that age itself is not the critical factor in determining to which group an elderly person belongs.

We are all familiar with pictures of the London Marathon showing seventy and eighty year old men and women competing: the "young old at 80". At the same time, you know the phrase "old before his time", denoting a relatively young person suddenly grown old, perhaps the "old old" at 50!

Mental illness

Growing old is quite a normal process. But it can involve becoming physically ill, for example with heart disease, or a stroke. Becoming mentally ill is not normal but is not uncommon in old age. The causes of physical and mental illness in old age are multiple, complex and complicated. Every older person with a mental health problem should have a full assessment, diagnosis, treatment and the chance to discuss their future care.

There are three broad areas of mental function that affect us all.

These include:

- Our mood (the medical term is "affect"): being happy, sad, anxious or agitated.
- Our cognition: remembering, feelings, thinking, understanding, learning and problem-solving.
- Our behaviour: the way in which we react, use our energies and perform tasks.

For the purpose of simplicity, mental illness can be divided into two main groups of disorders – organic and functional disorders. There is a danger however of becoming concerned about finding the right label or diagnosis. It is important that we consider each person as a unique individual, rather than a set of signs and symptoms.

Organic brain disorders

Features include:

- disorientation in time and place
- difficulty understanding
- difficulty concentrating
- difficulty remembering
- excitability and irritability,
- suspicion of surroundings and other people
- alternately sleepy and restless
- general lack of interest

You will notice that a number of these so-called "abnormal features of organic brain disease" are similar to some of the normal psychosocial changes which we noted previously as being characteristic of old age. It is very important to be clear that this is an illness, or group of illnesses, that have nothing to do with the normal process of ageing.

Causes

What causes organic brain disorders?

Acute organic brain disorders or confusional states are fairly common in older people. They may be caused by illness or the side-effects of drugs. A change in the social situation, bereavement or moving to a hospital or residential home may also cause acute confusional states.

Acute confusional states may be temporary or become permanent, dependent upon the cause. The priority is to find what is causing the confusion. In the majority of cases, treatment is successful once the cause has been found.

Chronic confusional states are usually permanent. The term dementia is used to describe conditions that result in the progressive loss of mental functions. The commonest form of dementia is **Alzheimer's disease.** It is responsible for approximately two thirds of the cases of dementia. It is usually a disease of old age but can occur rarely in people of all ages.

Multi-infarct dementia. This is the next most common cause of dementia. It is caused primarily by disease of the arteries, with a reduction in the blood and oxygen flow to the brain. The damage may be patchy, and depend upon which parts of the brain are first affected.

Parkinson's disease. A disorder characterised by trembling, a rigid posture, slow movements and a shuffling, unbalanced walk. The cause is obscure. Intellectual impairment can occur late in the disease. Dementia is very rare; if it occurs it is often mild at the outset, tends to become progressively worse. Sufferers often become depressed and withdrawn.

Huntingdon's Chorea. This is a rare, inherited disorder characterised by a complex pattern of rapid, involuntary, jerky movements, and dementia, which begins in adult life and is progressive – death occurring between ten and twenty years after onset. Suicide may occur in people suffering from this disease.

Trauma. Many organic brain diseases result from trauma or damage to the brain, for example the "Punch-drunk syndrome" which may affect boxers.

Drug or poison intoxication. Toxic confusional states, leading to permanent damage to the brain, may be brought about through use or over-use of a whole range of drugs, including alcohol.

Delirium Tremens (or "the DTs" as it is sometimes called) is the hallmark of the heavy drinker, and the fact that he can see "the pink elephant" when we cannot shows how his brain is being affected.

Vitamin B complex deficiencies and carbon monoxide poisoning also come into this group.

Infection. Infectious diseases give rise to brain disorder either directly by invading brain tissue, or indirectly through the production elsewhere in the body of toxins. Meningitis and syphilis are two classic examples.

HIV infection and AIDS related dementia Contrary to common belief, older people are at risk. They are sexual beings and some inject, or have injected, illicit drugs.

Tumours. The brain is one of the most common sites in the body for tumours. The resulting mental disorder will depend on the nature and location of the brain tumour.

Cause unknown

Turning now to the second main group of disorders associated with mental illness, we come to the functional disorders.

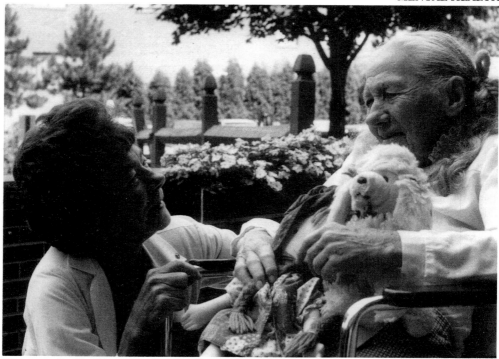

The mentally ill older person has double trouble, with the physical problems of old age too.

Functional mental illness is described as a group of disorders that have no physical cause. That does not mean that there is not a physical explanation, but simply that we are uncertain at present about the explanation for this type of illness. It is likely that this type of illness will always have been present, but may not always present itself until old age.

Before we look at what groups of disorders go to make up the functional psychoses, we must differentiate between *psychoses* and *neuroses*. For purposes of diagnosis, initially, each mental illness may be allocated to one of a list of major categories of disorder, which includes: psychoses, neuroses, drug abuse and personality disorder.

Psychosis is a mental disorder in which a person's mental capacity, affective (emotional) response, capacity to recognise reality, to communicate, and to relate to others, are impaired enough to interfere with their capacity to deal with the ordinary demands of life.

Neurosis is a mental disorder characterised by anxiety. The anxiety may be experienced and expressed directly, or indirectly through an unconscious psychic process. Although neuroses do not distort reality (unlike psychoses) they can be severe enough to interfere with a person's normal living.

Psychosis

The term psychosis includes the following main groups of disorders:

Schizophrenic syndromes
Schizophrenias in the elderly are marked by:

• disturbance in thinking, mood and behaviour

• hallucinations – a false sensory perception without a concrete external stimulus (seeing "the pink elephant" is an hallucination)

• delusions – a false fixed belief not in accord with one's intelligence and cultural background (a common delusion would be a person's expressed belief that they were Jesus Christ)

• being out of touch with reality.

Paranoid disorders

Paraphrenia is the name given to schizophrenia when it occurs for the first time in older age. Paranoid conditions may be mild or severe. It is important to remember that older people who have poor vision or hearing may be suspicious, but they are not necessarily paranoid.

From these symptoms it is clear that schizophrenia and paraphrenia are psychoses: sufferers are simply not in touch with reality. Elderly schizophrenics and paraphrenics respond well to drug treatment, but it should, of course, be carefully monitored.

Mood (affective) disorders

Mood-related, or "affective" symptoms seldom occur alone, but are much more likely to be associated with either physical illness or an event such as bereavement, the moving away of children, loss of status, retirement from a job. Affective disorders in the elderly usually have a better prognosis, the later the onset.

Depression

The majority of first depressive attacks, especially severe attacks, appear in the second half of life (between 55 and 65 in men, and 50 and 60 in women). Antidepressant drugs have been enormously valuable in combating depression. Depressive patients present with multiple symptoms, as follows:

• feelings of worthlessness, guilt, helplessness and hopelessness

• anxiety

• crying

• suicidal tendencies

• loss of interest in work and other activities

• impaired capacity to perform everyday social functions

• hypochondriasis

• anorexia

• weight change

• constipation

• headache

Hypomania

The other kind of affective disorder, mania or hypomania, is far less frequent than depression, especially in the elderly. Sufferers go to the opposite extreme of mood, on a "high" of energy and/or elation. Where it does occur it often follows a bout of depression, and responds well to drug treatment.

We tend to use words like "depressed" and "manic" in ordinary, everyday speech, to describe how we feel when we are either "down" or "up". In no way, however, should you confuse this ordinary use of these terms with the true depression and mania exhibited by psychiatric patients. There is absolutely no comparison: they are as different in kind as chalk and cheese. True depression can be so profound, and mania/hypomania so intense, as to render the sufferer psychotic, ie removed from reality and unable to cope with life.

Neurosis

The occurrence of neuroses in later life is far greater than that of psychotic breakdown. As mentioned above, neurotic conditions do not remove the sufferer from reality, nor do they totally disrupt his normal pattern of living.

A neurotic illness, however, can play havoc with a person's life, as we shall see in some of the following conditions:

Hypochondriasis

This is an especially common disorder in the elderly, characterised by a preoccupation with the organs of ingestion, digestion and evacuation, and with the heart and circulatory system.

Anxiety states

These are associated with increased muscular tension, difficulty in relaxation and sleeping, disturbances in the regular rhythm of the heart, gastrointestinal tract and urinary system disturbances, tremors, headaches, excessive perspiration, increased irritability, and a vague sense of impending doom.

Compulsive disorders

The compulsive person can be recognised by his over-conscientiousness, perfectionism, orderliness, over-attention to detail, and doubts about himself and his adequacy. Symptoms take the form of excessive cleanliness and orderliness, and endless and inflexible rituals to guard against mistakes, danger, etc.

Phobias

A phobia is an intense fear of an object or situation which the sufferer recognises has no real danger for him. There are many, many phobias, but the most common are "fear of streets and open places" – agoraphobia; "fear of crowded and enclosed places" – claustrophobia; "fear of high places" – acrophobia.

Most neurotic sufferers can be helped by therapy. The therapist must take into account that elderly people are generally slower to learn and adapt, but that apart, therapy can be very rewarding.

Double trouble

The older person with mental health needs has the worst of both worlds. They already experience the problems associated with normal ageing, things which are very familiar to us, arthritis for example.

In addition they have become mentally ill, an abnormal state in which they may experience a psychotic breakdown, like schizophrenia or depression, or some neurotic condition such as a compulsive disorder.

We have shown previously how this may affect the sufferer. Signs and symptoms have been given which show how they may be suffering medically, psychologically and socially.

Treatment will be available to help with these problems. The doctor will see to the patient's medical well-being, clinical psychologists and therapists of various kinds will attend to their psychological and social needs. If skilled nursing care is required, then trained nurses can provide that.

But, at the end of the day, the sufferer is just a person with many problems, not all of which can be dealt with by the professionals, no matter how good they may be.

It is the carer, whether they be informal (such as family/neighbours/friends) or formal (such as the care assistant) who has to deal with the whole person. As the person's problems increase at home, with perhaps more and more manifestations of mental illness, family and friends (the informal carers) reach a point where they can no longer cope.

The stress becomes too great for them to bear and, despite all the help and support which they are receiving, and despite all their care for and goodwill towards the patient, it may be essential for the well-being of all concerned to seek other types of care.

Coming into formal care, sooner or later, may be the answer to such difficulties. This is where you come in, as the care assistant/support worker. Providing the kind of support and help and care which a caring relative would provide is a good starting point, but the formal carer must go far beyond that level if he/she is to become an invaluable and fully integrated member of the team which will care for that older person for the rest of their life.

In the following pages, all the various aspects of the caring process will be examined with a view to providing you with the kind of information which you are going to need in order to do that job. The content is diverse and wide-ranging because the elderly mentally infirm person will have many and different problems.

As part of a training programme or on their own, the contents of this book will help you become a valuable member of the care team. You will be able to understand the difficulties of older people with mental illness and help them to cope with a life which may become increasingly more difficult, and about which they may understand less and less.

The better your knowledge, skills and attitudes are developed, the more you will be able to contribute to care and promote as much independence as is possible for every older person, caring for them in the widest possible sense.

Further Reading
Norman A (1982) *Mental Illness in Old Age: Meeting the Challenge.* Centre for Policy on Ageing.
Gearing B. Et Al. *Mental Health Problems In Old Age.* A Reader. Open University Press.

CHAPTER 2

How a good home can help

by Gwyn Roberts

No magic formula - caring is a challenge • To segregate or not • Imagine how it feels to be permanently confused • Helping residents stay in touch with reality • A safe and helpful environment • Communication, empathy and respect

Alzheimer's disease and senile dementia take their very heavy toll on all aspects of the daily life of the sufferer. Further on in this book you will find practical guidance and background information needed to promote the self-respect and wellbeing of the elderly mentally infirm people in your care. In this chapter I want to look at how the right environment can help, and how the right approach is vital.

There are no hard and fast rules about caring for an elderly person who is dementing; no magic formula that will suddenly make caring an easy and instantaneously successful task. Success comes over a period of time and comes from a philosophy, an attitude, a way of thinking. This I would summarise with one phrase: treat your confused residents as far as possible as though they were normal.

No one who provides care for the elderly mentally infirm will say that it is easy; some say it is frustrating and sometimes thankless because the person you are caring for is unlikely to show you any gratitude whatsoever for your hard work. What carers do admit, though, is that there is something special about this type of care that provides more challenge and job satisfaction than almost any other.

Unfortunately, now that we live longer, more of us are likely to become demented in our later years. It is also a sad fact that we, as sufferers, will be the only ones who may not understand what is happening to us. Confused elderly people have little or no insight into their situation, or at least if they do at the beginning, they gradually lose this insight as time goes on. It is often because of this lack of insight and the consequent danger that they may be in at home that they are the most likely elderly people to be placed in a care home, and the least able to understand why. Similarly, their lack of insight into the way they are behaving may put enormous pressures on families who are trying to cope at home, and lead to the final decision to "put Mum in a home" that Mum herself will never accept because she can't see the problem.

To segregate or not

There are not many homes in the country that specialise in caring for the elderly mentally infirm; most will now have a mixture of confused people and those who are perfectly aware of their surroundings but who have come into care because of physical difficulties.

This has led many experts to discuss the wisdom of segregating confused people (that is in separate units) or integrating them with mentally intact residents. At the present time, there is still no general agreement. The argument for integration seems to be that, in theory, if confused people are with "normal" people, their behaviour will be improved by example. There is some truth in this, in that social skills such as correct table manners can be retained for longer if everyone around is eating properly.

Unfortunately, this cannot be guaranteed and, in practical terms, what happens is that many "sensible" residents object strongly to having to spend time with those whose communication skills are deteriorating, whose eating habits may be becoming anti-social and who may well make inappropriate noises and be uninhibited in their behaviour.

My own view is that confused people should be "integrated" for as long as possible but that there should be opportunities for them to be segregated at times when their behaviour may present problems for others living around them. This means that they should have privacy when they are displaying anti-social behaviour; may eat at a table where their table manners will not cause disquiet to others and may spend quality time with carers who will sit and try to communicate.

It is sometimes the paid carer who will provide the only companionship that the confused resident craves. I have been involved in cases (not in homes in which I have worked) where confused residents have been confined to their rooms because the other residents have objected to their presence. This can lead to complete isolation unless the carers try to make provision for the individual to have a better quality of life.

Whatever we do as carers, we must ensure that the confused resident is not treated as some sort of sub-standard species. The quality of service that we offer to our confused residents should be no less than that offered to our mentally intact residents. While they may not be able to exercise quite the same range of choices about their lives, they should be given every opportunity to remain independent and live life with dignity.

Increasing confusion

Often elderly dementing people can seem to be demanding and difficult. When they come into a care home for the first time they have usually moved from home where their own possessions and surroundings have provided valuable clues to the world around them.

All the time elderly confused people are managing at home or with their families, they will be encouraged to stay there. It follows, then, that when they are admitted to a care home they are probably already becoming increasingly confused about things like the time of day, whether or not they have eaten recently, where the toilet is and indeed who the people around them are. It is possibly just these things that have triggered the decision to come into the home in the first place.

It is not surprising, then, that their reaction to a whole new set of circumstances is one of increased confusion and possibly agitation. Even after a period of settling in there is still the possibility of the resident becoming agitated and even a little aggressive when the things that are going on around them are making no sense.

One of the characteristics of dementia is a gradual disorientation: this means that the dementing person will not be able to place him or herself in reality. Although none of us with all our faculties can really imagine what that might be like, one could

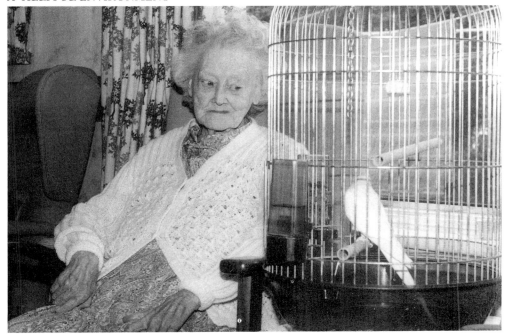

Residents should bring in as many of their belongings as possible - even some pets may be possible

perhaps think of being suddenly placed on a remote planet where day is night and night is day; where people around us talk in a language we have a vague recollection of knowing but which makes little sense now and where aliens seem to be in full charge of what we do. Perhaps in that situation if someone insisted we got undressed and had a bath, we might become a little aggressive too!

Orientation

All this confusion around and we, as carers, need to do something to help (if we are not to be viewed as aliens from outer space). First of all, it is important for confused people to be constantly reminded of reality, as this helps to make the maximum use of each resident's remaining faculties. When people have no real concept of time or place, it is very easy to become even more confused if the surroundings do not give consistent and accurate clues to what is going on. For example, there should be

easy-to-read clocks around – always telling the correct time.

Many homes have orientation boards which spell out the name and address of the home and a note of the state of the weather outside. I am not totally in favour of these because I think they can look very institutional if they are not designed properly. Also, there is a danger that staff take the boards for granted and stop talking to the residents about these simple facts. Nothing is as good as kindly and tolerant conversation to make residents feel in control of their lives.

Having said that, if it is possible to put up an orientation board that still retains a homely domestic look, then it is crucial that it is kept up to date. It is the greatest unfairness to residents who are already disorientated to give them information that is wrong.

A safe environment

Providing a safe environment must be a major consideration for anyone caring for a person with dementia. Potential dangers lurk everywhere. Elderly people are always at greater risk of having accidents than are the young because they are less agile, but with someone who is confused this risk increases. Judgement and insight into surroundings gradually disappears and deciding on the right action to take to avoid accidents can be completely impossible. For example, a kettle may be put on to boil with no water in it; or allowed to boil dry because the person has forgotten all about the tea he or she intended to make.

Rights and risk

Of course, the tendency then is to wrap the affected person in the proverbial cotton wool, just in case, but this is every bit as unacceptable. It must be remembered that dementing people are still thinking and reasoning – it is merely that these functions are impaired and become distorted. If carers take away all the risks that are endemic in everday life, they are leaving nothing behind for the dementing person to do for himself and thus taking away all his independence. So, how do we strike the balance?

Well, first of all, we should ensure that all the obvious dangers are minimised. Hazardous substances that the resident might drink should be locked away, open fires should be carefully guarded, tea-making facilities should be in a place where the resident can be easily supervised, etc. If carers look around for the sorts of dangers they would expect a child to encounter, and take precautions based on that, then they will be behaving sensibly.

Now I do not mean for one moment that the elderly confused should be treated like children. Clearly that is totally unacceptable, but I see nothing wrong with adopting a safety policy which is similar because I feel this puts caring for the elderly confused into perspective.

It helps if the physical surroundings are light and uncluttered. Pastel shades are more restful than harsh primary colours and can help towards a calm atmosphere. But it is important that rooms look like part of a home and not like an institution. Often the confused elderly person will be better able to cope with things that happen if they can recognise the decorations and furniture as being homely.

For this reason, it is also important that they have some of their own belongings in their bedrooms; it not only helps to make the rooms look more individual, it can also help jog memories that are gradually fading away.

Families should be asked to make up photograph albums of friends and relatives, all of which should be marked with names and relationships. Carers can then use these albums to talk to residents about people from their past lives who are important but who are becoming less familiar as time goes by.

Furnishing

Furnishing a home for dementia sufferers is a challenge. Upstairs windows must not open wide in case a resident decides to climb outside. Furniture should be functional as well as decorative and must be able to withstand a degree of mishandling. Wardrobes may need to be secured to walls so that they cannot be pulled down. The whole objective should be to make the home as safe as possible so that restrictions on residents' movement around the home are kept to an absolute minimum.

There used to be a tendency to provide plastic crockery for confused residents because glasses, cups etc. can easily be broken and thus create a danger. Thankfully this idea has now largely become outdated and domestic glasses and crockery are used more.

Indeed, setting a table and presenting meals as normally as possible may even have a positive benefit for confused residents since they are able to maintain correct eating habits for longer. Sadly, there will probably come a time when the dementing process has gone too far for activities like eating with a knife and fork to be remembered, but even then it is possible to make mealtime easier for the resident by providing a spoon instead. Taking over feeding is the last resort.

Good design

Some of the difficulties in caring for the elderly confused can be eased only if the home has been designed and built around their needs. For example, toilet facilities should be plentiful and in places where they are easily accessible to every resident. It is a sad fact that incontinence all too frequently becomes a part of the confused person's life, and yet this can be minimised if staff can set up a toileting regime that suits that individual and ensures that he or she is given the opportunity to be at the right place at the right time.

Unfortunately, many care homes have been converted from old houses and often there are not sufficient toilets around in the right places. There is little that carers can do about this problem if it exists, except to be aware of the need for regular reminding of where toilets are and the offer of help to get there at the right time.

Poor lighting may increase the risk of accidents as it may increase confusion. It is important that sufficient lighting is always available, particularly in landing areas at night when many confused elderly people tend to wander around. Obviously, blown light bulbs must be changed immediately.

The later chapters of this book will deal in detail with those aspects of the personality that are most commonly changed by dementia and how these can be handled by carers. But as an introduction to the subject, it might be useful to summarise some of these characteristics and look briefly at how the environment can affect the changes.

What time is it?

The fundamental change is, of course, loss of memory. This means that abilities and skills gradually become "unlearned" almost in the reverse order to that of a child learning those same skills. The skill of eating with a knife and fork mentioned above is a typical example of this.

It may seem strange, but often memories for things that happened many years ago remain intact, while what happened five minutes ago is forgotten. Therefore everything in the home must be geared towards jogging the failing memory for the things that are happening in the here and now.

It can, of course, be very frustrating to answer the same question over and over again in the course of a day, but a tolerant approach is vital. Remember that the resident has no recollection of having asked the question before. Sometimes distracting the person onto another subject or activity may help but there are no magic words to use that will help dementing people remember anything they said or did a few moments before.

Carers who work in homes where there are confused elderly people have to be extra tolerant and extra patient. Not all succeed, and if it is not something you believe you can do at every moment of your working day, perhaps you should not work in that environment at all.

When, where, who?

The second major change is that they become more and more disorientated. Time ceases to have any real meaning; the place in which they find themselves does not make sense and they may also begin to be unaware of who they themselves are. It is vital that residents are reminded of the "here and now" because without that information, the disorientation becomes worse.

It is difficult for us to imagine what this must be like but two examples of things that have certainly happened to me may ring a bell with you. I have often, when staying away from home, woken up in a strange bedroom and wondered (very briefly) where I am. Similarly when I have overslept (thankfully not too often), I have awoken with a jolt; completely confused for a few moments about what time, and what day it is. Imagine feeling like that at every moment of every day.

What can we do to help? Clocks that are always accurate and large enough for an elderly person to see are useful, as are calendars or a notice board in a prominent place showing, for example, a menu of the next meal or a topical comment about the season or the weather.

We should use the names of our residents constantly because this helps them to keep a sense of their own identity. But beware, it is important that an appropriate name is used. Nicknames and first names should only be used if it can reasonably be assumed that the resident would prefer that name if he or she had the ability to state an opinion. A mirror should be available in each room of the home so that confused residents can be given continual reminders of their own identity.

Communicating

A third change is one of communication. Words often become distorted or are simply forgotten; phrases are inappropriate and ideas cannot be transmitted.

It is important that we remember that talking is not the only way of communicating. Looking the person in the eyes while speaking, touching his or her hand, keeping still as you speak, can all help in effective communication, if only to make the resident feel important enough to be given your undivided attention.

A knowledge of the resident's past life sometimes helps the carer interpret the ideas he or she is trying to communicate. Writing things down may help. What is important is to recognise that a person who cannot easily form words and sentences may still comprehend what is being said. Carers should use simple phrases and sentences, and ask questions that may be answered with "yes" or "no".

Respect

The rest of this book is dedicated to the pursuit of excellence in caring for the elderly mentally confused. I have tried only to give a foretaste of the sorts of things one must be aware of in the environment that surrounds our residents.

Let us now look at some aspects of daily life in our care home:

• Are people encouraged to continue to feed themselves in an appropriate place, even if they have to use unconventional tools? *They should be.*

• Are they given their food on crockery that is pleasant and homely? *They should be.*

• Are their bedrooms nicely decorated with domestic-type fabrics and furniture? *They should be.*

• Are residents shaved in private and not in front of everyone else in a communal space? *They should be.*

• If residents are incontinent, are they led away with the minimum of fuss and changed in privacy? *They should be.*

• Are they dressed in clothing appropriate to their age? *They should be.*

Being old and confused does not mean people become something less than human. They are every bit as deserving of respect and privacy as anyone else. Remember that they cannot help themselves – you, the carer, must do it for them.

Points to remember

1. Treat your confused residents as though they were normal.

2. Confused people should have opportunities for privacy; to remain as independent as possible and to live life with dignity.

3. It is important for reality constantly to be reinforced. Everything in the home must be geared towards jogging the failing memory.

4. Dementing people are still thinking and reasoning; these functions merely become impaired and distorted.

5. Rooms should look like part of a home and not an institution. Residents should be encouraged to bring in some of their own belongings.

6. Being old and confused does not mean that people become something less than human.

7. Providing a safe environment must be a major consideration in caring for a person with dementia, because judgement and insight gradually disappear.

CHAPTER 3

Planning to care: from admission onwards

by Steve Goodwin

Making decisions • Take time and care over assessment
• Real people, real lives • The process of admission • Relatives - don't judge
• Close observation and records • Reality orientation and reminiscence • Care
of the very frail • When someone dies • Value yourself and your work

Throughout life most of us are involved in making major decisions that will affect not only ourselves but also those close to us. These may be decisions about employment, marriage, family matters, moving house, and later on retirement. Some of these are decisions that are forced on us by circumstance. In some we have a wide choice but in others little alternative seems apparent.

In older age the decision to move into a residential or nursing home or even a hospital continuing care facility is made, usually because of declining health and capability of the individual to support themselves or to be supported in their own home or that of their family. Whether the decline is gradual or sudden; whether the move is made highly reluctantly or quite willingly; the elderly individual should, wherever possible, be fully involved in the decision of whether and where to move.

For elderly people with a dementing illness, the ability to make this important decision may be well beyond them, particularly if we expect a yes/no answer. If a decision with or without them has been reached that they need to enter a home then it may be necessary to give them a trial period or gradual introduction to an establishment, perhaps through day care, to see if they can settle there. But for some elderly people with dementia even this may not prove useful, as any change from their normal environment may further affect their wellbeing or behaviour.

Assessment

Before any decision is made, there must be a thorough assessment not only of the elderly person and their capabilities, but taking into account all the circumstances, and what may happen in the future. This may seem quite complicated, and indeed it often is. But we must not forget or underestimate the great importance of this assessment. Just because the great move into a home seems inevitable, it will not necessarily be any less painful and distressing for an old person with dementia to give up their home or move away from family and familiar faces and places. Familiarity is often the anchor that has held that mixed-up and forgetful person, when tides of disorientation and confusion threatened to sweep them away from a near-normal existence.

What can make a move into a residential establishment less painful and distressing is good preparation for admission, and this begins at the assessment stage. Assessment is not just a one-off procedure, but should begin with an initial assessment completed where possible before admission. It is usual for one of the management team members, more often a qualified staff member, to undertake the initial assessment, but it is very valuable for a member of the care staff to be involved too.

The assessment should not be rushed, though often not a lot of time is available, especially if it has to be carried out for an urgent admission. A good assessment is much more than a "flying visit" where hasty impressions are made. The manager or trained staff may concentrate on business matters regarding the potential resident and may overlook important care issues that need to be highlighted. Some information may be very confidential or difficult to talk about. Maybe finances are involved or the elderly person displays anti-social behaviour that embarrasses relatives.

The circumstances may be quite tense: relatives may be tired out following months or years of continuous caring. Different relatives within the family may hold extreme or opposing views about the situation: one daughter may want their mother to go into a home, the other may not. All in all the need to tread carefully is important.

Assessment is equally about finding out what is *right* with the elderly person, even though they may have a severe dementia or be very handicapped physically. A balanced view is needed, incorporating the person's abilities as well as their handicaps.

Because we are only human we are very likely to make quick impressions and form hasty opinions. We need to focus tactfully on the facts: if for instance it is reported that the elderly person falls regularly, we must clarify why and when. Is it because their home has poor flooring? Is their footwear adequate? Is it just inside the house or when they are out as well? If incontinence is a reported problem area there may be some obvious factors in their present environment: they may have no commode, the toilet may be out of reach upstairs, they may be wearing too many layers of clothes which they cannot undo in time.

To add to the complexity of all this, the elderly person with dementia may not be able to give a reasonable account of themselves. Relatives or other carers may be distorting the facts through under- or over-estimating the problem, or even telling "mistruths" for many complex reasons.

A real person

If the initial assessment takes place in the elderly person's own home this can have added benefit for any care staff involved in the visit. It should help them see that this person is a real person with real, if often distorted, feelings, beliefs and values. The decor of the place, the photos and pictures, ornaments and furnishings, may gives clues to the kind of environment that helped that person feel at home. It should be possible for the person to bring some of those precious things into the home with them.

Care staff too should ensure that they come away from the assessment with key information that may help on admission. A simple tick list may be all that there is time to compile, but it should include information about mobility aids, dentures, spectacles and other less obvious issues: do they own a pet, attend clubs regularly, have a special friend or contact they would particularly miss?

Assessment is of course also a two-way process, not just asking endless questions but also an opportunity for the elderly person and their carers to speak and ask questions themselves. Again because time may be restricted, it may help if an information booklet is made available for relatives, describing the home and the process of admission, for them to read at their leisure. Perhaps the family may prefer also to fill background information in writing in their own time. This may give more time for important discussion while staff members are there with them face to face.

Care staff showing an understanding and tolerant approach to the difficulties and challenge involved in caring for elderly mentally ill individuals are more likely to obtain honest, open and useful information from relatives, and may make the process of admission that bit less threatening and disruptive for all parties concerned. First impressions count for a lot, but it is worth remembering that assessment is a continuous process, building on and reshaping the information. This is important in helping care staff to know residents better and to adapt and update skills, knowledge and approaches, matching them to the various and changing needs of elderly people with mental health problems.

Admission

In the process of admission, a lot more is taking place then just the home gaining another resident. The elderly person may be very anxious, more confused and disorientated than usual by the upheaval, and even from day one they will be feeling the bereavement of separation from home and family. Other confused residents may upset them; they may be feeling lost, afraid and very lonely. We may find this hard to believe when care staff are so friendly and helpful, their own little room is pleasant and cheerful and the other residents so chatty and jovial. Surely they should be pleased to have so many new friends their own age to talk to?

Before one of the care staff is tempted to reassure them with the highly dubious statement, "This is your new home" they should first reflect on what they are implying, or trying to achieve with those familiar words. It may be extremely difficult, if not impossible, for that elderly confused person to make a new home anywhere, however comfortable, homely and well-planned the environment. They may well live there for the rest of their life. Whether they will ever consider it home, however, is a matter for much discussion, and discussion in these matters is very important for all staff.

Not all elderly people with dementia react adversely to admission, however. Some can settle down right away, though problems may arise later. The sense of loss and upset of moving may not strike until weeks or months after admission.

Welcoming

The kind of reception a new resident is given may well greatly affect their acceptance of and ability to settle in the home. It is always nice to feel that you are expected, to see a familiar face and feel welcomed. The confused elderly person may feel more assured and less anxious if staff know a little about them, their family and past history. The first hour or so may be best spent quietly with a member of staff or a relative, just having a drink of tea, especially if they are agitated or the home is a bit noisy or busy.

It is very important that the new resident is made familiar with the whereabouts of the toilet right away. A long car journey, the effects of medication, and a feeling of anxiety could all make the use of a toilet an urgent priority and an incontinent accident could be hugely upsetting for the elderly person and their relatives.

Relatives

The relatives or past carers of the new resident may need just as much if not more care, understanding and reassurance on the day of admission and the all-important following days. They may have enormous doubts, feelings of guilt and also be feeling quite anxious, afraid and lonely themselves. After all, this may be the first time they have been separated from each other. A spouse or daughter of the new resident may well be returning to an empty house themselves. Just because a carer could no longer manage does not mean to say they no longer wanted to manage.

The mixture of emotions involved on the first day of admission could be very complicated and again the need to tread carefully is very important. Care staff can help by asking for support from the relatives and not presuming that they will take over fully now. The day of admission should not be seen as a "takeover" but the beginning of shared care where relatives continue to play a key role. Relatives and other carers must not be seen as an awkward by-product of residential care, but right from the earliest days be encouraged to remain involved. Not all care staff or relatives will find this easy – probably because it isn't easy – but the effort it takes to make it work, even with unpopular and apparently over-zealous relatives, will prove worthwhile. Lasting damage can be caused if staff jump to wrong conclusions about relatives as well as residents.

Settling in

Not all residents will be able to have a room of their own, not all may want one anyway. Whether they are sharing or not they will need to be settled into their room, and their belongings unpacked. If they want to they can help with this, directing where things should go and how they like their clothes kept. Of course some residents may be adamant that they are not staying, that they have to "get home". There is no point in arguing with them or causing further upset, so it may be best to leave the case until later, returning when they are more amenable or later on when they feel tired.

A consistent and honest approach is needed with elderly people who are forgetful and confused, but it is important also not to antagonise them unnecessarily. All staff and relatives will need to know that this is the approach that is being used. It would not be helpful or kind in the long run to tell an elderly person reluctant to stay the night that they could go home in the morning just so that they would go to bed, if indeed they were going to be a permanent resident in the home. Although in the short term it may solve the staff's problem, it may only add to the resident's confusion, and it doesn't build up trust.

Helping an elderly confused resident settle in a home may take weeks or months, therefore a plan of care needs to aim at balancing long term goals with tackling immediate problems. This very often means having to prompt residents constantly that they no longer live at their previous address, they now reside in a nursing or rest home, and even remind them that their wife or husband died many years before.

Close attention

Being admitted into a busy home or hospital can be quite a traumatic experience, especially if an elderly person is used to living alone or with just one or two other people. Imagine the change of having to live with perhaps as many as 20 or 30 others. For anyone this would be expecting a great deal; for very confused people it can be even more difficult.

It is always helpful if the staff involved in

the initial assessment are about for the first day of admission, but as this is not always possible, it is important that other staff have read and discussed any background information and the assessment report. All this will help on the first day of admission.

If a new resident is known to be prone to aggressive outbursts, for example, extra care will be needed to keep them away from particularly noisy and disruptive residents, especially during the first few days. They may be recognised as a wanderer, so you must record the clothing they are wearing and observe them closely. Staff may need to take it in turns to stay with them.

Because staff numbers are often short, particularly during early evening and mealtimes, this may be a good time for a relative to help out on the admission day. If the new resident is sharing a room at night, it is helpful to introduce them to the sharer early in the day, so that any potential problems can be ironed out and, you hope, a future relationship nurtured.

It is likely that the first day of admission will be a testing one for all concerned. Even if a new resident appears to be settling, they should not just be left to get on with it. Time throughout the day should be spen on a one to one basis with staff away somewhere quiet, even if only for five minutes, so that both parties can get to know each other better. It also gives the resident a little solitude to gather their thoughts, establish the basic details of where they are, why they are there and what happens next. After all, they may just have spent the last 30 minutes talking to another resident who told them that we're all in prison and the staff stole all their money.

It is usually the care staff who have most contact with residents, so the information they feed back in either written or verbal reports is crucial to ongoing assessment. Close observation on the first days of admission, accurate reporting and the recording of positive as well as negative aspects of behaviour are all important.

During the first night it would be only natural for the resident not to sleep well. It will be a different bed (unless they have brought their own), a different room, a different person perhaps sharing. The home may be quieter or noisier than they are used to. Any night report needs to take account of this, and any change in sleeping tablets should be avoided for the first couple of weeks until a fuller review can take place and other alternatives considered. Relatives may be able to advise about sleeping habits; the resident may have had a disturbed sleeping habit for a long time – they may have worked shifts or night duty for many years. A good assessment will reveal these things.

The important thing about the first day of admission is to keep an open mind and not to be too swayed by strange behaviour of the elderly individual. Throughout the following days the consistent, patient, and enthusiastic approach needs to be maintained by staff. The resident can be more gradually introduced into the activities of the home, spending more time with other residents. But there should still be quiet periods, opportunities for staff to keep prompting in general conversation where the elderly person is, what is happening with their relatives , and reminders about the time of day and the date.

Reality orientation

This procedure of trying to keep confused residents in touch with factual truths about their circumstances and practical information to help them with their immediate environment, is known as reality orientation. Sometimes special boards are used to indicate the day, date and season or weather conditions, placed where they can be seen by all patients. Clocks with large faces so even visually impaired elderly people can

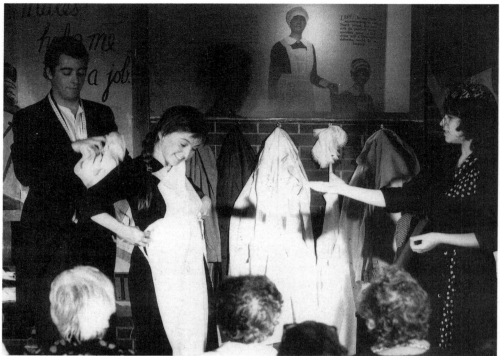

Above and facing page: Actors recreate bygone days for an audience of elderly people.

see them are sited around the building so residents are reminded of the time of day. It is essential of course that these clocks and calendars are kept accurate, otherwise they add to confusion and disorientation.

To help confused or forgetful elderly people find their way around the home, doors can be marked with their appropriate description. This may help an elderly person with dementia identify a toilet rather than having to try several similar looking doors and being incontinent in the process. Signs need to be large enough to see at a distance, sited low enough to be in the visual range of old people with restricted head movement, and yet look as normal as possible in a homely environment.

The principles of reality orientation can be taken much further. Residents can be encouraged to remember other people's names by staff wearing name badges; footprints could be printed on the floor to guide residents to toilets. Regular group sessions with staff and residents can be used to try and establish wider information about the real world in which they live, and their previous history. This aspect of looking back into the past with residents and recalling the times with which the elderly mentally frail are mostly more familiar, merges into the practice of reminiscence therapy.

Reminiscence

Reminiscence is something we all do, whether old or young; it is a natural and often enjoyable aspect of human behaviour. Elderly people with dementia-type disorders usually have a better recall and memory of events and information from many years ago than they have of quite recent events. They can often recall who they sat next to at school, but find it difficult to bring to mind when they had their last meal or what they ate.

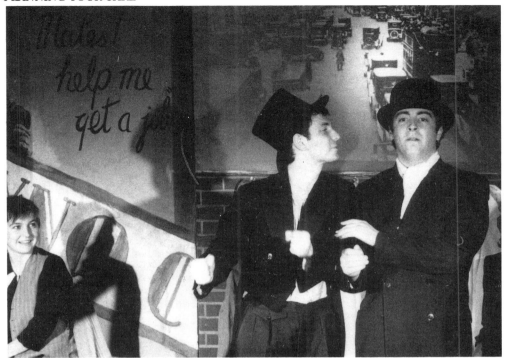

Age Exchange Theatre specialises in reminiscence therapy for elderly mentally infirm people.

We need to keep elderly people with dementia in the real world, so that they can be seen as real people who deserve and expect the same rights, standards and human needs as everyone else, and are valued as individuals of worth and status. Reminiscence helps them recall the significance of their past lives, and it helps staff and others reflect that they are still the same person who held down a job, raised a family, went away to war or campaigned for better prospects for themselves and others, including the young care staff of today.

An elderly lady resident, now frail and much ravaged by a severe dementia, can otherwise easily be overlooked and devalued as just one more elderly statistic, grey and uninteresting.

People's histories and experiences should never be denied or confiscated once they enter a care setting or develop dementia. Old photographs can be used as evidence that life has taken place and that

we need to value such individuals as real people with a place in the real world. If we value people with dementia, then quite simply we will find it easier to respect their rights and maintain high standards of care.

Reminiscence sessions can be made more interesting and conversation stimulated by the use of props such as old photographs, newspapers, memorabilia from past decades, music and singalongs from forgotten eras. It is important to remember however that some people's memories are not all happy; some are very painful and private. People aged 80 and over have lived through two world wars; there is a great deal of poverty and bereavement among the happy recollections in their treasury of memories.

Both reality orientation and reminiscence are useful, indeed essential, aspects of care for people with dementia. Recognising their history and the experiences of past lives will help care staff see that these events have helped shape the beliefs, opportunities and expectations, and influenced the circumstances of these elderly individuals today. They should be regularly considered and used in daily practice by care staff. This is best implemented by building them into each resident's individual care plan.

Care plans

During the first few days of admission an individual care plan should be developed. This is a written plan of care that sets out the purpose of that resident being in the home, and a broad outline of their overall needs, highlighting problem areas and focussing on what the main aims of care will be in these areas. Care goals will need to be defined, as well as suggestions made on how to achieve them.

This important piece of work must not just be a paper exercise that makes interesting reading but which staff find unusable, irrelevant and unworkable. Therefore the best approach will be a simple, clearly understandable and practical plan. On most occasions a trained member of staff or one of the management team is responsible for the formulating of the care plan, but it is very important that care staff and where possible relatives and other interested parties do contribute.

The first draft of a care plan can only really be a sketch, until a clearer, fuller picture of the new resident can be drawn. The plan will need to be regularly discussed and reviewed, and any necessary modifications developed into the next phase of the care plan.

Like the assessment reports, some aspects of the contents may be confidential or need special consideration. A resident may have particularly difficult behavioural problems. There may have been marital problems before the onset of the dementia, other family upsets may be relevant.

These may need the help and consideration of the wider family and yet at the same time be very difficult to raise or discuss.

Confidentiality, accuracy and privacy all need to be key considerations in writing and evaluating care plans as well as in day to day reporting by care staff. Some relatives may wish to contribute to reports or care plan review meetings. This may help care staff to consider more carefully what they are feeding back about residents and their families and ensure that they can justify their comments and get facts straight rather than often loosely formed opinions.

Care plans can help new staff and temporary staff get a quick overall picture of the main aims of care for each particular resident. It can also highlight special considerations and the best way of tackling problems or difficult behaviour. The care plan therefore provides a constructive and creative approach which could otherwise be overlooked, especially when residents are badly affected by dementia and other disabilities. A good care plan doesn't just focus on problem areas, but also draws the attention of care staff to what individual residents enjoy doing, what motivates them and what can be done to halt a decline when general inprovement is no longer expected.

A working plan

So that all staff are aware of what each individual resident's care plan is all about, and so that it is read and used as the framework for each day's care practice, it needs to be at hand. This may mean in each person's bedroom, or in the office, but it must be accessible to appropriate people. (Staff should discuss who is "appropriate" for confidentiality's sake). Wherever it is kept, staff should regularly refer to it. It will need to be reviewed regularly, and the date and type of review due should be built into the care plan, so that it doesn't get overlooked or avoided.

Care plans should focus on what is right about each elderly mentally frail individual as well as what is wrong with them. They should use information where appropriate from the person's past life and experience to help point towards present circumstances and future care goals. The care plan also needs to give consideration to the broad range of needs that such elderly people have, not just the mental and physical aspects of their health but their social and psychological needs, and the important spiritual needs, often overlooked with this client group.

The care plan is not a clever sounding compilation of well-meaning intentions. It is a plan of action in which all staff are involved, that builds upon the day to day assessment and observation of care staff and other professionals and family. It is often the care map that care staff need to refer to when they feel they are lost, are going astray from time to time with a resident or when there seems little point in the very existence of certain residents as the progress of dementia becomes more rapid and quality of life seems completely absent.

Physical and mental frailty

Many elderly people with dementia have other complicated disorders, as most of them in residential or hospital care are aged 80 and over. If arthritic or other joint or mobility disorders are also present then pain may cause regular problems. An old, mentally frail person may not complain of this but instead become more withdrawn, or agitated and aggressive, especially if they are walked or moved by care staff too hastily or carelessly.

Other physical disorders may be worsened by the person's mental decline. An elderly gentlemen who is a constant wanderer may soon become exhausted or collapse if he has congestive heart disease or other coronary or respiratory conditions. The use of sedative drugs may further affect his overall wellbeing. A simultaneous decline in physical and mental health is sometimes seen as an individual ages. On the other hand there are many very mentally frail residents who remain physically strong, active and reasonably fit into their 80s and 90s.

Sadly for many elderly people with dementia, especially Alzheimer's disease, the later stages of their illness often bring a severe decline in overall health, and usually a dramatic decline in quality of life. For anyone closely involved with the elderly person, especially their family, this period can be an emotionally painful experience when it seems little can be done medically to counteract the decline that is so clearly seen.

Care staff too may be saddened as they daily witness the distress of such human experience. After all most would dread ever ending up in such circumstances themselves or seeing their own family or friends decline in this way. These natural feelings, however, should not distract them from the enormous challenge and important role they can play in salvaging the best quality of life possible for such individuals. It is important not to underestimate the good that can be done, and the value of each carer's own personal involvement.

Skilled care

There are unfortunately still misguided staff about who believe that caring for such individuals is like looking after babies, or that all such people need is tender loving care. It is sometimes true that the level of care needed will incorporate feeding, changing clothing, toileting, washing, bathing and careful positioning in chair or bed. It is also true perhaps that all this should be done with a great deal of tender loving care and attention.

What cannot be overlooked, however, is that care staff are handling real people who have had very real lives and who have real feelings and emotions. They have the same right to expect dignity and respect as any other grandparent or senior citizen. The ability to exercise those rights will however often rest in the hands of the carers who are continuously involved and who must never lose sight of these things even in daily routine practices.

Tender loving care is important but without skilful judgement, relevant knowledge and insight, it will not alone really help an elderly person who is in severe pain or dehydrated. Good care staff will always be on the lookout to note changes in residents and record observations so that more than tea and sympathy is offered when urgent nursing or medical intervention is needed.

Daily care

Care staff can make the daily practice of care more pleasant for even the most severely handicapped or frail resident. A bath, essential to maintain hygiene and good skin condition especially for the regularly incontinent resident, enjoys the warm water then a longer soak may be comforting. Perhaps massage or aromatherapy could be used to good effect, or hydrotherapy if facilities are available.

Selecting the correct chair and bed will be a vital step for residents who are immobile without staff help, and all staff will need to know about pressure area care to avoid such residents developing sores from sitting or lying in one position for too long. Sometimes pressure sores are too readily accepted as inevitable with such elderly frail people. The pain , discomfort and danger of widening infection caused by such a sore cannot be overestimated.

Food and drink

Diet can also affect skin condition and proneness to tissue breakdown, so not only the amount of food we give residents is important but also its nutritional value. Care staff can help maintain quality of life in this area too by ensuring that food given to residents who need feeding or who are on special diets is of good quality and nicely presented. It may need to be kept warm , as feeding residents can be time consuming and should never be rushed. Care staff may need to plead this cause with managers so that adequate staff are available at meal times.

Elderly people with eating or swallowing difficulties may soon become malnourished and dehydrated, if they are not getting sufficient nutrition and fluid. Nobody, with or without dementia, should have to drink tea or eat food once it has gone cold.

Keeping a frail resident comfortable will help maintain their quality of life. Being comfortable involves consideration being given to their total environment: this means the temperature of the room, clothing not being restrictive, environment not too noisy, no foul smells, suitable bed or chair, a pleasant and stimulating outlook that changes from time to time, a place that feels secure and safe and where other faces and voices are reassuring and express genuine commitment and consideration.

There may be a special treatments or pastimes that please such elderly frail residents, that we can build into their care plan and the staff's daily practice. Perhaps music is such a factor, or a dog or children visiting; it may be certain foods or chocolates and cakes, being outdoors in the garden or the sensation of water in the bath or pool. Things like this can make a seemingly hopeless existance more purposeful and pleasant.

It may be that for some a certain hymn or passage of Scripture is significant and meaningful; we cannot tell at what level every individual may function, what they can understand, how much of what goes on around them filters in.

Death

Finally, when death does occur, it may be widely described as a relief and a blessing. But this does not always make the pain and grief caused to close family and others any less than any other death in the family. Even though expected, death brings much sorrow; this may extend to care staff too, who often have a close and personal involvement with the elderly individual and their family. It is therefore only right and natural that staff should be encouraged to grieve too, and share their feelings with the family.

Value your work

It sounds as if everything a member of the care staff says or does in caring for such elderly individuals is important and complicated. Certainly in the busy rush of daily care practice it would be unrealistic to ask all staff to sit down and consider every aspect of their behaviour and actions before they started each duty. What does need to be considered by each member of the care staff, however, is that the job they do is extremely important and often goes unthanked. The pay is often poor, the work certainly testing and physically and emotionally demanding. Even the best staff, who feel valued themselves and who value the work they do and the people they care for, will never be perfect. They will however be giving near to the best that they can, which can be improved on with better training and facilities.

Staff involved in caring for elderly people with dementia are often only introduced to the individual following the onset of their illness. They see perhaps a person who is old, grey haired, confused and unsteady on the shifting sands of reality. How much of what is seen is that person's true self and how much distortion for better or worse is due to dementia, cannot easily be measured. But each member of the care staff must ensure that they are always treated as real people in a real but equally changing world.

Points to remember

1. Assessment is continuous and involves considering what is right with the individual as well as what is wrong.
2. In a shared approach to care, relatives have a right to be involved. See them as a positive resource. Don't pass judgement - they may have other trials and responsibilities.
3. Reality has many sharp edges but people with dementia can face change and realities, especially if they are to be maintained in a real world.
4. Living with large groups of other people in close quarters is not really natural. Don't be surprised at conflicts, problems and stresses.
5. People with dementia are unique individuals who need to maintain a personal continuity between the past, present and future.
6. People with dementia have the same human value as anyone else and are entitled to respect and dignity, and to be seen as people of worth and status.
7. Good quality of care relies heavily on good care staff. Accurate reporting, an open mind and a keen eye will help others help you to help the patient.
8. When death occurs it often casts fear and sadness around. Dying without pain, in peace and surrounded by family and close associates is a very positive achievement.
9. The good that no one sees us do is usually the best. In your self-appraisal remember to congratulate yourself every now and then, and remember your colleagues too!

CHAPTER 4

Talking and listening

by Karen Bryan and Jane Maxim

What is communication? • Problems with sight or hearing
• Language difficulties • Confusion and dementia • What to say and how
to listen • Encouraging conversation and relationships

Talking to elderly mentally infirm people is perhaps the most difficult aspect of care to get right. We can talk to them, but do they listen? And if they do listen how much do they understand?

This chapter looks at how elderly people communicate and the differences between elderly people with a number of specific conditions which can affect communication.

We then go on to suggest ways of making communication easier, and we have divided this part of the chapter into two parts. One looks at general principles which are helpful when talking and listening to an elderly mentally infirm person, and the second part explores ways in which carers can help these people to communicate.

What does communication involve?

Communication is a process of conveying information between two or more people. Communication involves talking, listening, writing and reading.

Before communicating there needs to be a thought, which is then put into words and sentences to convey meaning. The words are spoken using coordinated movements of the larynx, tongue and face to produce speech. But part of the message is usually conveyed by other means:

– hand and body movements to produce gestures, like shrugging the shoulders
– changes in voice and pitch, for example we describe someone as "sounding" angry
– the use of facial expression, like a smile or a frown.

The listener needs to listen to the actual words spoken as well as attending to the other information that the speaker is conveying, in order to fully appreciate the meaning. So listening involves using your eyes as well as your ears.

Being able to communicate with other people is a vital part of our lives. For many elderly people it is particularly important because limitation in mobility can restrict their daily activities.

For mentally infirm people, communication may be made more difficult by mental deterioration and resulting changes in behaviour. Before considering these changes however, it is useful to look at the effects on communication of normal ageing and specific diseases. These may add to the elderly mentally infirm person's problems with thought, memory and other mental operations.

Mental ageing

The process of ageing usually causes people to slow down, so that talking and understanding may be slower than in younger people. Older people also have occasional difficulty in finding the word they want. This is known as the "tip of the tongue state" and happens to all of us sometimes. They also show differences in their style of talking. They may tend to give lots of details and perhaps even "ramble" a little.

But these changes in style of communication do not affect their everyday ability to communicate. It is therefore important that elderly people are given every encouragement to talk and to express their opinions. A lively, interesting environment will help to stimulate conversation.

Sensory problems

Many elderly people have difficulties in hearing and seeing. These problems can interfere with communication so it is vital that hearing aids and spectacles are prescribed, regularly worn and regularly cleaned. The elderly mentally infirm person with a poor memory will need to be reminded every day about wearing and using these items.

Some older people do not like wearing a hearing aid. An alternative which can be used for any resident consists of a microphone attached to a small amplifier. You speak into the microphone and hold the amplifier to the resident's ear. Most equipment catalogues for the disabled advertise these useful aids and they are relatively inexpensive.

Teeth are very important for clear, understandable speech. Many elderly people have badly fitting dentures or do not wear them, usually because ill fitting dentures cause discomfort and even pain.

The importance of attending to eyes, ears and teeth cannot be stressed enough. Imagine yourself trying to have a conversation while wearing another person's glasses, with cotton wool in your ears and a large moving object in your mouth. Try it and you may gain some insight into the problems that many elderly people have to cope with!

Is the resident
- wearing cleaned glasses?
- wearing a hearing aid in good working order?
- wearing dentures which fit well?

Language difficulties

As well as the sensory problems of hearing loss and poor sight, certain specific problems can affect communication:

- dysphasia
- dysarthria
- depression
- confusion

Dysphasia

This is a disturbance of the ability to produce or understand language, which may affect understanding, speech, reading and writing. The most common cause of dysphasia is a stroke affecting the left side of the brain. Many people with dysphasia also have some paralysis on the right side of their body but some do not, and these people, without any physical symptoms, are sometimes wrongly diagnosed as having some form of dementia.

Residents who enter a home for the elderly mentally infirm may have had a previous stroke causing dysphasia. In general the communication abilities of dysphasic people do not deteriorate, and some may show improvement if given suitable encouragement.

People with dysphasia have difficulty in producing speech. For example they might say "tea" meaning "I'd like a cup of tea" or "di" to mean dinner. Sometimes the person may make an error of sound, eg "do" for "no"; or a word error, eg "man" for "woman" or "he" for "she". Sometimes understanding can be well preserved despite the person's difficulty in speaking.

In other dysphasic people, speech is very fluent but not many specific words are used so very little information is conveyed. For example: "Oh, yes, well you know, it's all very well, never mind". Someone with this type of "empty" speech may also have great difficulty in understanding what is said to them.

When trying to communicate with a dysphasic person, observe what the person can and can't do. Try to note what is happening when the person does manage to communicate, so that you can provide effective help. The following general guidelines are helpful to remember when speaking to a dysphasic person:

1. Slow down your rate of speech.

2. Remove distractions such as television, which will interfere with listening.

3. Break down your speech so that you give one part of a message at a time.

4. Try to imagine what the person might want to say: using questions that only need a yes/no answer may be useful. For example: "Do you want to have a wash?"

5. Give the person time to speak and answer.

6. Maintain contact with the person while they struggle: look towards them, look interested and wait patiently.

7. Show sympathy if the person becomes upset or frustrated.

8. Remember the person is not stupid: speaking very loudly and very slowly does not help. Use your normal voice and expression.

9. Ask the person's opinion.

10. Use gestures while you speak, and look out for their gestures and facial expression. For example, a person who mixes up "yes" and "no" will usually show which they mean by their facial expression.

11. Remember that speech is a great effort; do not expect a dysphasic person to talk for too long, and be alert to signs of fatigue.

> • Dysphasic people are very aware of what is going on around them.
> • Try to talk to them as normally as possible.
> • Show sympathy if they become frustrated when talking.

Dysarthria

In dysarthria the nerve supply to the muscles used in speech is disrupted, so that production of speech is difficult. The muscles may be weak and floppy, making speech jerky with sudden changes in loudness or pitch. Muscles can also be unco-ordinated, causing speech to vary unexpectedly. This variation can cause the dysarthric person to sound slurred or even drunk.

Dysarthria does not affect understanding of language or the ability to decide what you want to say. There is also no disruption to reading and writing skills unless there are other physical problems such as poor eyesight or weakness in the hand and arm muscles.

When communicating with a dysarthric person, it is important to allow them time to speak, to listen carefully and to watch for gesture and facial expression. It is often the case that people in everyday contact with a dysarthric person can "tune in" to their speech and understand them very well.

For some dysarthric people very little speech can be produced or their speech is unintelligible. It may be possible for the person to use writing, a communication chart or an electronic aid to help their speech or even replace it. You may need to contact a speech therapist to discuss what is needed for that person.

Depression

A significant nymber of elderly people suffer depression. Depression can profoundly affect communication, particularly the will to communicate. As well as showing little interest in events and their surroundings, the depressed elderly person may not start conversations or respond when spoken to. Their speech will often be very quiet, with no variation in voice or expression.

All these aspects of depression may give the impression that the person is not able to communicate properly. Give the person time to communicate and accept whatever form of communication the person chooses. If you ask a question and they respond by nodding, then respond positively to that nod.

Emotional impact

It is important to consider the impact on an elderly person of not being able to communicate normally:

• difficulty in expressing immediate wants, for example to go to the toilet

• difficulty in expressing feelings such as sadness, anger

• difficulty in expressing needs, for example to see a family member or write a will

That this leads to immense frustration is understandable, but it often gains the person the label of "difficult". Communication difficulty also affects relationships with other people, family, carers and friends, and can lead to social isolation.

What does communication difficulty mean?
Difficulty in:
expressing immediate wants
expressing feelings
expressing wishes

Confusion

Confusion can be due to acute problems such as urinary tract infection, sudden admission to hospital or a drug side effect. Confusion may also arise as part of a more chronic mental deterioration or dementia.

Communication is affected by confusion in the following ways:

– reduced recognition, understanding of and response to the environment
– difficulty with recent and distant memory
– inability to think clearly
– disorientation to time, place and person

However confusion does not usually affect vocabulary, the ability to form a sentence or produce clear speech. Where confusion is due to an acute event, the resident should be treated appropriately for the underlying cause. Once they begin to improve they need to be helped out of the confusion by talking about where they are and what has happened. The resident will also need lots of reassurance and encouragement to help them to start communicating appropriately again.

Dementia and communication

The vast majority of people in residential homes for the elderly mentally infirm will be suffering from a dementing condition which progressively impairs all aspects of their mental functioning, including the cognitive skills necessary for communicating. The exact pattern of mental deterioration will depend on the cause of dementia, its progression and the interacting effects of any other problems that an elderly person might have, for example hearing loss and poor eyesight.

The combination of mental deterioration and deafness is a particular problem. An elderly person may mishear and then have the added problems of not fully undestanding what they have heard.

An elderly woman may be asked "Would you like your hair done?" She responds by saying "no" and tries to push the speaker away. Her facial expression shows her to be frightened. If she also has difficulty in speaking she may not be able to explain why she is frightened or ask what was said to her. So her feelings of fear and frustration may increase, leading to unexpected or even violent behaviour.

There is a particular pattern of communication difficulty recognised in dementia which leads to the following problems:

• confusion and disorientation so that the person is less and less aware of what is happening around them

• decreasing memory ability with a tendency to forget recent things and dwell on the past

• loss of the ability to understand, seen in inability to draw "obvious" conclusions, difficulty in putting together different aspects of meaning

• the person becomes unable to cope with any form of indirect meaning and therefore what they say and think becomes very concrete (so they cannot understand jokes, for example)

• loss of the ability to reason by talking things through in their own minds

• difficulty in using language to explain anything, with a tendency never to reach the central point of what they want to say. As dementia progresses the elderly person will be less and less able to achieve meaningful communication, but steps can be taken to help residents make the best use of their remaining skills. They need:

• stimulation – so encourage social situations which provide good opportunities for communication

• positive measures to promote **orientation** to people, time and places

• an **interesting environment** with events happening that give residents something to talk about

• control over their own activities, as far as possible, and the possibility of making **choices**, for example over meals, activities and visits.

Residents can be assessed by your local speech therapy service. Even if treatment is not appropriate the speech therapist can advise you on how best to communicate.

Communicating

Communicating with the resident who has any form of dementia is a challenge, and your approach does depend very much on how far the dementia has progressed. Before we discuss how to talk to the affected person it is useful to consider how dementia progresses and what aspects of communication are still possible at different stages.

Stage 1. At times the person may seem bewildered when you speak to them. They may say that they are having difficulty remembering people's names or a specific word that they want. They may also seem depressed and avoid certain tasks which remind them that they can't do all the things they could in the past.

Stage 2. The person now has more difficulty with orientation to time, place and person but they are better in familiar surroundings. Their speech may now be very vague or consist of a familiar "story" that they repeat over and over again. They may talk about their parents as if they are still alive. Understanding simple language is still possible.

Stage 3. The person now probably says very little or may have a particular phrase that they use a lot. One lady whose language skills were followed over several years, used the phrase "shopping centre". Sometimes swear words can become the recurrent phrase, but they are not being used in the same way that we would use them.

Finally the mentally frail person will stop talking and will not be able to understand any language. At this stage they are often bedridden and in need of complete nursing care.

To discuss communicating with the elderly mentally infirm person we will divide talking into three areas:

• conveying a specific message

• conveying a general message

• helping communications.

Preparing for communication

How can we best convey a specific message? In the first and second stages of dementia it is usually still possible to convey specific messages if we prepare the resident in the right way.

1. Face the person and make eye contact on the same level as the resident: sit if they are sitting, stand if they are standing.
2. Use their name *before* you begin speaking, to make sure they are attending.
3. It may help to use their name from time to time in the conversation and to touch them on the arm or hand to remind them to listen.
4. Keep any background noise or distracting activities to a minimum (turn down the TV).

The person may have difficulty both in understanding what is said to them, and in talking themselves. This means that any form of conversation is difficult for them. When we talk with another person, we usually look at them and use words which indicate that we are addressing that person. It is very important to make sure the resident is ready to listen or to talk. It is often quite noticeable that people with dementia do not look at the person talking to them. It is as if they have forgotten that this is one of the rules of conversation.

Another of the rules of conversation is that if you start off a particular topic, unless you indicate that the other person can change the topic, the other person will continue it. People with dementia often violate this rule. They may know that they should respond to what you have said but they have not understood what has been said to them. You comment that the weather looks lovely today. Mrs B says that she wants to go home and where are her shoes? She has responded to your conversational opening but she has probably not understood what you have said.

Even when the resident does talk to you, it may be difficult or impossible to understand what they say. Residents who have had strokes may have particular difficulty in getting across what they want to say but, unlike the person with dementia, the dysphasic resident may know exactly what it is they want to say and may try a variety of ways to get their message across.

If you listen closely to what the resident says, often the form of a sentence is quite normal and the words are in the right order, but it is specific words which are not right. In the early stages of dementia only a few words may be affected. Perhaps the person cannot remember names very well and uses pronouns (he, she, they) instead of the correct name. This can be very confusing; you may need to ask a question, for example "Did Jane come to see you?"

Sometimes the wrong word may be used but it may be close to the right word – "I want my eyes" instead of "I want my glasses" The person may call everyone by the name of a close relative or insist that you are a relative.

Sometimes it is possible to build up a web of meaning to help the person. They may not understand one specific word, even if it is repeated, but if several words or ideas are used that have similar meanings or are all to do with the same topic, then understanding may be helped.

What to say

Here is an example of a carer talking to a resident first thing in the morning and trying to help that person orientate themselves to the time of day:

Mrs Jones, good morning.
Did you have a good night's sleep?
It's time to get up now.
You can get dressed and then you can have your breakfast.

Here is another example of a carer talking to a resident about her son:

Mrs Jones, your son Tim has just rung.
Tim is coming to see you tomorrow.
It is Friday today and tomorrow, on Saturday,

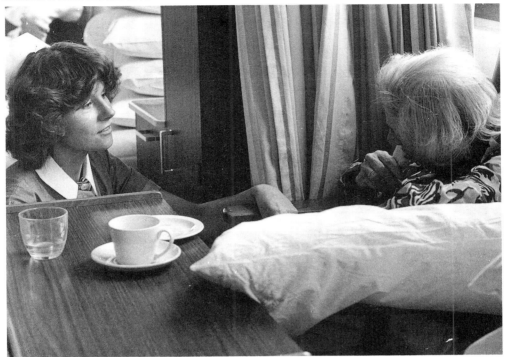

Good communication: always face the person and make eye contact.

your son Tim is coming here.

Note that the carer has used the son's name, Tim, rather than "he".

Sometimes it is useful to use a forced choice. First introduce the topic and then give the person the choice.

Would you like a drink, Mrs Jones?
Would you like tea or coffee?

How to listen

Misunderstandings can happen between residents and carers quite easily. Try to work out what the basic message might be and don't take what has been said as exactly what the person wanted to say. Above all don't react with abuse if you are verbally abused, however hard it may be to stop yourself. The resident will usually calm down much more quickly if you speak calmly and gently.

As an example of listening to the under-lying message we will consider the resident who says that something of theirs has been stolen. They may mean that it is missing, or that it has been moved, or even that they are confused about what is happening.

After we had visited an elderly man at home, he complained to his daughter that the speech therapist had said he was "going senile". She had visited him at home where she found a very suspicious elderly man with a severe hearing loss. She explained in words and writing why she was visiting him but he was obviously depressed and frustrated by his disabilities, and in fact was worried that he was becoming senile. His complaint was his way of voicing his concerns.

Coping with verbal abuse:
- Speak calmly and gently
- Think about what the person may really be trying to say
- Don't contradict

In early stages of dementia, when the person may be aware that their ability to function and think is changing, they may be depressed about these changes. If that person is already a resident in a home, they will need particular care and reassurance at this time.

Getting the message across

In the later stages of dementia the person may not understand the specific words that are being used, but you can convey a general message. This message is conveyed not by what you say but how you say it. The resident may well be able to pick up the emotional content of the message through the rhythm of your speech. You can put across sympathy, anger or firmness just by the tone of your voice.

This point may be particularly important if you have any residents in your home for whom English is not the first language, and if there are no carers who can speak the person's language. Facial expression and tone of voice can convey a great deal, although they cannot, of course, be as good as a carer who does speak the relevant language.

One elderly woman we know has great difficulty in understanding and following a conversation but sits entranced by game shows on the television. We think that she is responding to the excitement of the compere's voice, the participants' body language and the clapping of the audience.

Another woman had retained her ability to act appropriately in a social situation. She would always ask how we were, would we like to sit down and comment on how well we were looking. Sometimes she would make a comment which was appropriate for that person, commenting on dress or their hair. She sounded interested in our conversation even when she obviously did not understand it. She also responded to changes in our tone of voice very quickly. And when we laughed, so did she.

Helping conversation

When a new resident enters a home, it is a good idea to make a record of some of that person's characteristics. Was the person noisy or quiet, solitary or gregarious? What are or were their interests and hobbies? What is their past job and life history? It is particularly important to take the first and last names of spouses and relatives either from residents themselves or their relatives. Then when they begin to talk about "Tom", everyone will know whether he is a son, husband or just an old friend.

A good way to stimulate conversation is by using memories from the past, photographs or music for example. But do remember that not everyone will like or respond in the same way to the same music. You may like country and western but do they?

Can any of the residents play the piano? It is quite possible for people to retain their musical skills until at least stage 2 of dementia.

Familiar TV programmes or old films can also be useful but only if they are watched actively. The resident needs to be orientated to that particular programme. Switch off when the commercials come on. Just as we are sometimes caught out and it takes us a few seconds to realise that the commercials have begun, the person with dementia will find this change even more confusing.

Some residents may understand the radio better than the TV while others find that the sound and pictures together on TV give more clues to what is going on. If someone has been a keen film goer then they may react with great pleasure to old films, but you may need to find out who their favourite film stars are.

How can you help when a conversation is started? Because it is difficult for the resident to understand, it is better for you to pick up the topic of conversation from what they say. While trying to get an elderly lady to eat, she said she didn't know who the food belonged to, and should she take a chance? We said: "Take a chance. Go on. Take a chance. The food looks good. It's your food". She then said "Alright. I'll take a chance".

What about helping residents to talk to each other? It often seems as if residents avoid talking to each other but this is not really so. Communication takes place for all kinds of reasons: because we work with someone, find an interest in common, or they are our family and we want to share our thoughts.

The resident may be in surroundings which seem unfamiliar because of the memory problems they have. The people who do talk to them most are the care staff so the person naturally learns to respond to that care and interest. It may need your intervention to start conversations between residents, and it is much more easy to start conversations when there is some activity going on. Chapter 13 will give you plenty of ideas but remember that activities for more than two or three residents need very careful planning.

Points to remember

1. Make eye contact when talking.

2. Ask simple yes/no questions to help clarify what the person is saying.

3. Make sure you sound interested in what the person is saying.

4. If the resident needs them, make sure they are wearing clean spectacles, hearing aid in working order, dentures which fit well.

5. Communication difficulty means the resident is not able to say what they want or how they feel.

6. The elderly mentally infirm person needs your interest and encouragement to talk.

7. They need help with understanding where they are, who you are and what time of day it is.

8. Social events give residents something to talk about.

9. Giving the person choice over their own activities, food and visits can help to maintain good communication.

10. Coping with verbal abuse can be difficult. Speak calmly and gently.

CHAPTER 5

Managing disruptive behaviour

by Michael Maltby

Describe the problem clearly and exactly • Look for reasons and ask about the past • Can the problem be prevented or tolerated? • Behaviour modification as the next option • Violet - a case example

The aim of this chapter is to offer some general guidance on coping with disturbed and disruptive behaviour. Unfortunately there are rarely any "quick-fix" solutions to behavioural problems. Just because one thing worked with Mrs X does not guarantee it will work with Mr Y!

The only practical way to proceed is to take a step back to assess each situation as fully as possible. Different approaches can then be considered and tried. Even if an effective solution is discovered it will need to be reviewed as circumstances change.

This is essentially a problem-solving process which has to be gone through as each problem arises. In this chapter are some ideas to consider as you work through the main steps listed below:
1. Define what the problem is.
2. Look for any possible causes.
3. Decide what action to take.
4. Take action and evaluate progress.

This is a general approach to follow which can be applied to many situations. It is not possible to go into every behaviour or situation in detail. The specific problems posed by aggression, wandering and incontinence are dealt with in later chapters.

Defining the problem

It is useful to distinguish between:

(a) those things which a person used to do for themselves but can no longer do
and
(b) those things which some "confused" people may start to do, perhaps for the first time.

To most old people it is what they can't do that is the problem. Being unable to follow a conversation, manage your own affairs or even dress yourself properly can be a source of distress and indignity. However, for those of us offering care, the problem often seems to be what the person starts doing for the first time.

For example, the previously compliant person may start to hit out, resisting all practical help. A quiet well mannered person may shout and scream for no apparent reason. Another person may start interfering with other people's things, perhaps hiding their own possessions and accusing others of theft.

It is important to keep these problems in perspective. In particular to remember that the problem is not the elderly person themselves but what they do. It is easy to label people as "difficult" or "anti-social" but this is usually misleading and unhelpful. Very few people, if any, are difficult or anti-social all of the time. However it can seem that way if we label them in those terms and ignore evidence of other more acceptable behaviour.

Perhaps the most positive thing to do is to recognise that all so-called difficult or anti-social behaviour is really a problem of management. It therefore represents a challenge to us to find the best way of coping. This avoids labelling the person and makes our task clearer: to respond to the challenge without ignoring the other needs of the person.

No list of such "challenging" behaviour can be complete but some common examples are identified below:

- verbal rudeness, demands and accusations
- repetitive questions and actions
- screaming and shouting
- extreme emotional outbursts and over-reactions
- night-time disturbance/restlessness
- agitation and interference
- hiding and hoarding things
- physical aggression
- self-injuring behaviour
- inappropriate toileting
- wandering
- uninhibited sexual behaviour

In practice every problem is different and so must be assessed individually. One way of going about this assessment is to ask a series of questions about the behaviour. For example:

WHAT exactly happens?
WHEN does it occur and for *HOW* long?
WHERE does it occur?
WHO is it a problem for?
HOW is it a problem for them?

When trying to define a problem in detail in this way it is important to avoid general statements, such as: "He is difficult at meal times". What is needed is an exact description of the behaviour that occurs and its effects on other people. For example:

"Mr Smith always eats his breakfast quickly and then gets up from his table and takes food from Mrs Jones who is blind and eats slowly. Mrs Jones gets cross and screams out but she can't stop Mr Smith.

This upsets the staff on duty who can't always keep a close eye on Mr Smith while serving the food. The problem rarely occurs at other meal times or with anyone other than Mrs Jones."

It may be useful to go through the questions together with everyone involved in the person's care to try and build up a complete picture. Sometimes the results can be quite surprising. A problem that at first seemed huge can be reduced to manageable proportions when you look at it more closely. Perhaps other people don't see it as a problem at all, or have found a way of coping with it.

Looking for reasons

After arriving at a clear description of the behaviour, it is worth trying to understand what the reasons for it might be. This is by no means an easy task. By its very nature, "confusion" in elderly people can make full understanding difficult and sometimes impossible.

In fact you don't need to understand the problem completely before you act. However the understanding you have is likely to influence what you do, and the way you do it, a great deal.

To blame a person for the way they behave achieves very little and often gets in the way of understanding why they act as they do. This does not mean people should be treated as entirely irresponsible, but the reasons for their behaviour need to be considered first. The behaviour may be the only way a need can be expressed, or may reflect something about the *situation* which is wrong, rather than the person.

Among the factors which can contribute to challenging behaviour are:
i) changes in mental functioning.
ii) physical and sensory difficulties.
iii) social and emotional reactions.

Mental changes

Perhaps the most obvious of these is loss of memory. This might be the straightforward reason why someone keeps asking the same question again and again or forgets where they put something.

Some changes are more subtle but can be just as problematic. For example lack of the ability to comprehend language may cause someone to misinterpret what is said and act inappropriately. Some people seem to lose the ability to monitor their own behaviour, so they act on impulse without regard to the consequences.

More dramatic still is the effect of unrealistic beliefs or "delusions" which some people may act on. For example, the belief that other people are after their things may cause a person to hide property, or to lash out at anyone who comes too close.

Physical and sensory difficulties

The effects of pain and physical discomfort can often be masked in an elderly person who can no longer communicate clearly. Instead they may come out as agitated or unsettled behaviour or sometimes as shouting and screaming.

Undetected problems of eyesight and hearing can increase confusion and disturbed behaviour, particularly in an unfamiliar environment. In fact the environment itself can contribute to some problems if it is unsafe, confusing or uncomfortable. The person who strips off their clothes may have no sexual motives but simply feel too hot sitting by a powerful radiator!

Social and emotional reactions

Most people have a strong need to relate to other people and this fact considerably influences their behaviour. As adults we expect to do this with a degree of independence and self-respect. The situation of an elderly "confused" person can be seen as both depriving and threatening in this repect. They have often already lost many of the significant people in their lives and may also have lost control of their own affairs. An awareness of this situation and their own failings can stimulate strong emotional reactions. In the early stages extreme emotional outbursts, sometimes called "catastrophic reactions", can occur as people catch a glimpse of what is happening to them.

Later they may tend to withdraw from social demands or become aggressively independent in an attempt to retain some limited control over their lives. It can be frightening to accept your own needs and trust people to meet them. Far safer, maybe, to resist help and blame others for everything that is going wrong, or alternatively to withdraw completely into your own world.

Ask about the past

Light can sometimes be shone on individual situations by finding out more about a person's previous behaviour from friends and relatives. Current behaviour may be an exaggeration of past patterns or an expression of a particular individual's established needs or fears.

A useful practical approach to any specific behavioural problem is to try and establish if there are any triggers which set if off, or anything that follows it which may

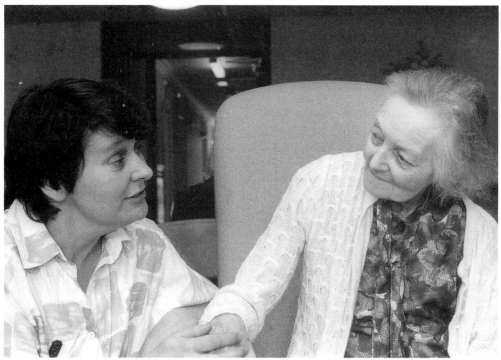

Encouraging a person's orientation and sense of belonging helps to reduce disruptive behaviour.

make it more likely to happen again. This can be done in the form of an A B C analysis of behaviour where:

A = the Activating event or situation
B = the Behaviour
C = the Consequences that follow

Simply keep a note or think through what happens immediately before the behaviour arises, and what happens immediately afterwards. Does the person get a lot of attention for their behaviour (C), or always react to a certain member of staff (A)? If any pattern emerges, this can go a long way to explaining the behaviour and gives a clue as to what could be done either to avoid or minimise it.

Deciding what to do

Broadly speaking there are three different strategies that can be adopted in the face of challenging behaviour:

i) Prevention
ii) Toleration
iii) Modification

The first of these is obviously the best. If the problem can be prevented from happening, or at least minimised, everyone is better off. It may be that a problem which can't be prevented can be coped with by making a few adjustments to the pattern of care. Only if prevention or toleration fail should emphasis be placed on trying to change or modify the behaviour itself.

Prevention
Much of what can be done to prevent or minimize challenging behaviour is simply standard good practice in the care of elderly people. Listed below are some of the factors which can make the biggest difference to people who display behavioural problems.

• Maintain NORMAL EXPECTATIONS. What you expect a person to do influences the way they actually behave. Look for the best from someone and you are more likely to get it.

• Compensate for MENTAL DISABILITIES. Good care involves helping people with what they can't do for themselves. With physical problems this is usually obvious but mental disabilities can easily be ignored. Anything which helps a person's orientation and sense of belonging is likely to help reduce disruptive behaviour. Using names on doors or labels and signs along corridors can help. Remembering to use strategies of Reality Orientation in conversation will also help settle many people.

• Encourage INDEPENDENCE and ACTIVITY. It is often easier to do things for a confused person than let them attempt things themselves. It can also seem very hard to engage them in constructive activity. Unfortunately this can result in frustration and a complete lack of purpose for the elderly person which may fuel inappropriate attempts at activity and independence. Try to get them to do small things for themselves and engage in short periods of activity with other people.

• Avoid any form of PROVOCATION. This may seem very obvious but is all too easy when time is short and patience is wearing thin. Perhaps the single most important thing is to allow time when you approach someone to tune into *their* state of mind. A calm unhurried approach which makes a person feel you are trying to understand them, is ideal.

Toleration

Not all behaviour can be tolerated, but in many circumstances it may be possible to accept it, as long as it does not actually cause anybody any harm. Many forms of sexual behaviour fall into this category. Contrary to popular belief most older people retain their capacity for sexual enjoyment. Inappropriate and disinhibited behaviour may pose problems. However, if the individual has some privacy it need not be unduly disruptive.

Noisy behaviour at night can sometimes be put up with by a careful choice of room, or if rooms are shared, by someone who is hard of hearing!

What is not acceptable is to cope with a person's behaviour by physically restraining them in any permanent way. This is an infringement on the person's freedom. Even in an emergency it is usually better to distract someone, rather than try to restrain them with any use of force.

Some behaviours are so difficult that it may have to be agreed for someone to move elsewhere. This should not be seen as a sign of failure. Some places are more suitable than others for tolerating and coping with particular problems.

Modification

Some forms of behaviour can be changed or made more manageable by the use of drugs, particularly tranquillizers. However these drugs often have unwanted side-effects, and many people are unhappy about taking them. It would seem preferable to try other methods first and to maintain these efforts even when medication is also being used.

Before seeing if it is possible to modify a behaviour, it is necessary to carry out an ABC analysis of the behaviour as described earlier. From this analysis, two possibilities may emerge for changing the behaviour:

a) *Altering the activating event or situation (A).* If any event or situation seems to trigger the behaviour regularly, efforts can be made to change the triggering circumstances. Alternatively, a problem may only arise in a certain context, or at a certain time of day, and therefore can be anticipated more easily.

In the example given earlier, where Mr Smith took Mrs Jones' food at breakfast, the trigger could be that Mr Smith has an empty plate and is still hungry. Anticipating this, he could be given a larger portion or a second helping, which might avoid his anti-social behaviour towards Mrs Jones.

b) Altering the consequences that follow the behaviour (C).

This is a deceptively simple thing to do but can be very effective if practised consistently. Many behaviours are maintained by what happens in response to them. For example it is not uncommon for someone to obtain quite a lot of attention for their difficult behaviour. This can be quite rewarding for someone who otherwise might get only limited attention from anyone. In other situations a person may be given cigarettes or food to try and stop them behaving badly. In the long term this is likely to have just the opposite effect!

In fact a behaviour might be repeated again and again just because of the rewarding consequences that sometimes follow it. If this is the case, it can pay to minimise any attention given to the behaviour. This will only work if everyone responds in the same way.

An effort should also be made to provide the reward at another time, when the person is behaving in a more appropriate or acceptable way. If you simply ignore a person's behaviour they are likely to behave increasingly badly to get what they want from you. The idea is to provide the attention, or whatever else they want and need, but only when they are behaving acceptably.

A word should be said about trying to use any form of punishment to alter someone's behaviour. Don't. Apart from being unethical, it is a totally ineffective strategy with most confused people. The emphasis should be on rewarding appropriate behaviour wherever possible.

Taking action

It is often easier to have an idea about what could be done about a behavioural problem than to turn this idea into a plan of action. Every member of staff can try things out for themselves, but this is unlikely to be fully effective unless other people are taking a similar approach. The key is to try and involve as many people as possible at each stage of the problem-solving process. This helps to generate a lot of ideas and means you can agree a realistic plan to follow.

You can rarely expect quick results from anything you try to do. In fact behaviour can sometimes seem temporarily worse when established patterns of care are altered. For this reason it is important to give anything you try a fair chance to work before rejecting it. However, at the end of the day the best approach is to experiment. Try things out and learn from your own experience what works best.

Any measure of success depends on what you are trying to achieve. If your aim is to find ways of making a behaviour more tolerable you wouldn't expect it to go away, but you might hope to reduce its effect on other people. A preventative approach hasn't failed just because some problems still occur. The best you can hope for is to decrease them.

Similarly behavioural modification shouldn't be assessed only in terms of the elimination of unwanted behaviours. Any increase in more constructive or appropriate activity indicates considerable success.

With more complex problems, it is well worth trying to keep a written record of the problem and any action taken. This need not be elaborate. A few regular notes or a daily chart is usually sufficient. You can learn a lot about a problem in this way and get a much clearer idea about the effects of what you are doing. It is also helpful to set a date in advance when progress can be reviewed. This gives you something to aim for and ensures that new action can be taken if necessary.

Help and support

With some behavioural problems, the point is reached when professional help may be required to assist with the situation. In addition to the GP, specialist services are increasingly available. These can offer medical and psychological advice on the management of challenging behaviour in elderly people.

It is important to recognise the need for support. Few things are so stressful and emotionally exhausting as caring for people with persistent behavioural problems. Nobody has limitless patience. It is natural to feel angry and upset when your efforts to care for someone are often frustrated. It is all too easy to cope with this by treating some people with less consideration than others. Alternatively your own health can suffer as you struggle to maintain high standards.

The only sensible thing to do is to try and recognise your own feelings. If possible have the courage to be open about them with others. You will usually find other people have experienced something similar and can be a source of support. You can't really expect to care for people whose behaviour is difficult unless you take some time to care for yourself. Chapter 12 explains how you can do this.

Violet - a case example

Violet Smith had been a popular resident. She had been in the home for about two years. Although sometimes a little confused, she used to recall the past in detail and loved talking to people. However over the last six months her behaviour had gradually become more of a problem.

At first she just seemed to lose interest in the TV and radio. Then she became more difficult to talk to. Finally she began to shout out for no apparent reason, much to the annoyance of other residents. The more the staff did to try to understand what she wanted the more she shouted, until one day in fury another resident hit her.

The staff wondered whether Violet's hearing might be the problem or whether she had deteriorated mentally. They arranged for assessment which confirmed a significant hearing loss. Tests of mental function showed no further deterioration in memory but found that Violet had developed a problem in understanding and using language. As a result Violet was provided with a hearing aid and staff took increased care to help her communicate.

Violet's behaviour improved. She showed a renewed interest in the TV and radio but still shouted out when they were switched off. The staff decided to monitor her behaviour and found that she only shouted when she had nothing to listen to or occupy herself with. She stopped as soon as someone talked to her. In fact some of the staff would even sit with her when she shouted to stop her upsetting other people.

The staff realised that although her poor hearing and lack of understanding was the original cause of her shouting it now continued as a means of getting much needed personal contact and stimulation. As an experiment they agreed to only give her personal attention when she was *not* shouting but to do this whenever they could. In addition someone had the bright idea of letting her use a personal cassette player to listen to her favourite music without disturbing other residents.

The results pleased everyone including Violet. She gradually stopped shouting as she found it actually prevented people talking to her. In addition she obtained great pleasure from listening to music in a way she had never experienced before.

Points to remember

1. Try to see the behaviour as a challenge, rather than the person as a problem.

2. Define the behaviour with care. Ask: what, when, where, who, how?

3. Consider carefully what the reasons for the behaviour might be. Take note of mental changes, physical difficulties and social or emotional factors.

4. Remember that prevention is better than cure. So maintain normal expectations, compensate for disabilities, encourage independent activity and avoid provocation.

5. Try carrying out an ABC analysis of the behaviour where:

A = the Activating event
B = the Behaviour
C = the Consequences that follow.

6. See if it is possible to change any trigger (A) or any rewarding consequences (C) that follow the behaviour.

7. Make an effort to reward appropriate behaviour wherever you can, for example with attention.

8. Before taking any action involve as many people as you can, and try to take a consistent approach.

9. Try things out, and learn from experience what works best by monitoring the results.

10. Recognise the difficulty of the task. In particular be aware of your own feelings and the need for support.

CHAPTER 6

Aggression and violence

by Alan Higson

*How do we define violent behaviour? • Understanding the causes
of frustration, the roots of aggression • What to do when violence erupts
• Taking stock and learning after the event*

T he word "violence" is over-used
and misunderstood in our society
today. It conjures up instant
pictures in our mind, making us run away
either physically or mentally. A violent
storm makes us fear for our safety. So does
the knowledge that one of our clients is
likely to behave violently. Violence is
something that we all fear, yet we are all
potentially capable of demonstrating it.

What is violence?

So what do we mean when we talk about
violence and aggression? The two words
are often used together but do they mean
the same thing? Is aggression a mild form
of violence? Or is it the threat of violence?

There are as many definitions of what
constitutes violence as there are theories of
what causes it. Most people would agree
that murder is a violent act, but is suicide?
Both result in the death of an individual.
The throwing of a punch by one person
against another with the intention to hurt
or cause injury is usually described as violent
behaviour. But what of a boxing match: is
that sport or violence? Shouting and swearing may be anti-social, but are they violent?

The environment in which an act takes
place has a bearing upon the way that it is
perceived. Each society determines what it

will, or will not, tolerate as acceptable behaviour. Behaviour that is perfectly acceptable in a
psychiatric hospital may not be tolerated in a
Five Star Hotel. Carrying a gun in the High Street
of any British town would result in severe
repercussions, but could be perfectly acceptable in other countries. Things that you do in
your own home may not be acceptable in the
homes of friends or relatives.

The dictionary defines aggression as "the
first act of hostility" and violence as "excessive, unrestrained or unjustifiable force".
But who is to determine what is, or is not,
excessive or unjustifiable?

For our purposes, let us define *violence* as
"behaviour directed to cause harm, damage
or injury" by physical force, and *aggression* as
"a feeling likely to lead to violent behaviour". Aggression and violence can then be
seen as a continuum, with aggressive feelings
possibly leading to violent behaviour.

If this is so, what is it that causes people
to feel aggressive? One theory is that *frustration* is the cause of violent behaviour.
This gives us a model:

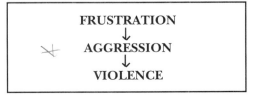

FRUSTRATION
↓
AGGRESSION
↓
VIOLENCE

With such a model in mind, we can see there are various points at which we, as carers, can attempt to intervene. We may be able to stop frustration leading to aggressive feelings, or aggression leading to violent actions.

Frustration

Ask yourself how you would react to being told that you couldn't behave in your normal way, now that you were living in a communal home. Rules had been set on meal times, times of getting up or going to bed and standards of dress. Decisions like when to have a bath, watch television or leave the home, were no longer yours to make.

Would you feel upset, annoyed or even angry? What if you had to share a room with someone else, especially if you did not like them very much? Other people always telling you *what* to do, *when* to do it and *how* to do it; people half or even a quarter of your age.

Can you begin to imagine the frustration that you would feel if you had no control over your own life? If you had no privacy. If rules were imposed upon you, often without an explanation. If you needed help to perform basic acts of living like dressing, washing and going to the toilet. If the only time that anybody touched you was to help with these. If you had no one to talk to. If there was no one for whom you were special. Would you feel frustrated, angry or aggressive?

By recognising that people want to be involved in decisions that affect them, and play a part in controlling their own lives, we as carers can begin to eliminate the frustrations that may lead to a violent incident. Every person for whom we care is an individual and wants to be treated as such. The lack of choice is de-humanising. If you treat someone as incapable of controlling their lives, can they be blamed for not controlling their emotions and becoming aggressive or violent?

But we must not forget that there may be physical reasons for the aggression. Certain drugs, both prescribed and illicit, may cause an aggressive reaction. So will some medical conditions. Elderly people often become very agitated and aggressive when they are constipated, for example.

Aggression

Aggression often occurs when people are unable to communicate feelings in more appropriate ways.

People demonstrate these aggressive feelings in many ways. Some ways are more obvious: shouting, swearing, banging doors, pounding the table or stamping the feet. Others begin to cry. For some people the signs are less obvious: they may become very white, begin clenching their fist, they may start to shake or perspire, they may begin foot tapping.

The signs are all associated with fear, and the "fight or flight" syndrome. When an individual feels threatened, either physically or mentally, this "fight or flight" defence system comes into operation. They either run away from the situation or fight against it. This running away may be by physically removing themselves from the environment or mentally denying the reality of the situation.

It is important to remember that in nearly every aggressive situation, the aggressor is afraid. A person who is afraid can also be dangerous. In order to avoid violent behaviour, or a physical attack, the aggressor's fear needs to be overcome and their aggression dissipated. In order to manage the situation you also need to overcome your fear. It is normal to be afraid when confronted with an aggressive and potentially violent situation as no one wants to be attacked. Whether you are of slight build or built like a tank, it is natural to be afraid of physical harm.

As a carer, it is important to appear calm and not aggravate the situation by losing your self-control through fear. But it is very difficult to remain objective and rational when you are afraid. The "fight or flight" syndrome applies to you as well and must be overcome in order to defuse the situation. Fear is contagious: if you allow your fear to be seen by an aggressor through your body language, they will become more afraid. This will make you more fearful and so on until violence starts.

If an aggressor does not see you as a threat then there is a greater chance of their fear subsiding; then you will be able to discuss the situation rationally and so avert violence. It is perfectly reasonable to tell your client that you are feeling afraid of him. By stating the fact, you are already dissipating your fear and not letting it build up. You are also able to continue to think logically.

If the client starts to express aggressive feelings in words — even shouting and swearing — you should encourage them and accept the feelings. Don't try to defend the situation that is causing the aggressive feelings, or you will aggravate the violence by getting into a struggle of wills.

Your client should be encouraged to look for other ways of resolving any inner conflict. The philosopher Plato said that mental conflict was self-initiated. If an individual chose to be hurt by what was said or done to him then he would be hurt. But if he chose to say that the word or deed was of no importance then he would be unaffected by it. However, you should never judge somebody for what they feel. Feelings are neither right nor wrong. Everybody has an absolute right to their feelings and only the behaviour that they demonstrate, what they do, can be judged.

It may be that a thoughtless word or deed by a member of staff, perhaps you, has caused the aggressive feelings. Perhaps a sincere apology will be enough to calm the situation. It may be possible to assure that the cause of the frustration will be removed, but you should never do this and then go back on your word. You must be honest and open with your client. If the situation cannot be changed then do not say otherwise.

The client should be sure that you care about them and their feelings. Most people who have lost control of their feelings welcome some control and order being restored. A concerned carer who restores calm and control will be valued by the angry client. If you have confidence in your ability to calm the situation and show no impatience or anger, this will assist in defusing the situation.

Time is on your side, unless someone is in imminent danger from the situation. Use good eye contact and listen actively to what you client is telling you. Your reactions can make the difference between calm being restored and violence erupting.

Violence

If a violent attack does occur, it must be dealt with quickly and professionally. The priority must be to avoid injury to anyone, including the violent client. However, never attempt to manage the situation on your own. Ensure that you summon help before any restraint is attempted. Shout, sound an alarm, get to a telephone, anything to ensure that help will come. If you are overpowered or injured before you can raise the alarm, other clients may be in danger without anyone realising what is happening.

You may need to break away from a client who is holding you, in order to summon assistance. This must be done in such a way as to not cause injury or an escalation of violence, and therefore the degree of force should be the minimum required to manage the incident. This "minimum use of force" applies to both breaking away from an attack and restraining a client from an attack.

Both the severity of the attack and the age of an attacker should be taken into account when considering what this minimum force actually means. Greater force will usually be required when restraining a young person than when restraining an elderly client, although this is not always true and care should be taken when assessing the situation.

You must always decide with your colleagues what your course of action is going to be. It is no use running in to hold a violent patient and then asking what you are going to do. Each person involved must know the entire plan: how the restraint will be applied; who will do what; when to apply restraint; and where the client is to be taken for recovery. This plan should be decided upon well in advance of its being needed.

If a carer is working in an environment where violent behaviour is not uncommon, it is advisable that they receive training through an approved "Control and restraint", course.

It is not possible to describe the techniques of control and restraint here, as it is only by practising them that safety can be ensured. Courses usually include techniques for breaking away from an attack, in order to summon help, and the techniques of restraining a violent client and removing them to a safe place for continuing care.

In conclusion, it should always be remembered that a violent client is as deserving of your care as any other. You should neither ignore nor over-react to a violent situation; your job is to manage it as calmly and efficiently as possible.

Incidents should be used as a learning situation for all those involved, both staff and clients who managed, or who witnessed, the occurrence. For many onlookers, the incident may have been a very frightening experience. The feelings of all those involved should be discussed. Staff should discuss the situation openly, without recrimination, to explore how the incident could have been avoided, and the manner in which it was ultimately managed. In this way, our individual experiences may be shared and some future aggressive and violent situations may be avoided.

Points to remember

1. Frustration may lead a client to feel aggressive.
2. Aggressive feelings can lead to violent behaviour.
3. Violent behaviour must be managed, not just allowed to happen.
4. The carer should actively look for and remove any possible causes of frustration for the client.
5. An aggressive person should be encouraged to express anger verbally and avoid a violent incident.
6. Try to appear calm and if possible discuss the situation.
7. Avoid defending situations or making promises that you cannot keep.
8. When a violent incident does occur, never attempt to deal with the situation alone. Always call for assistance.
9. Keep restraint to the minimum.
10. Encourage staff and clients to share feelings after such an incident.

CHAPTER 7

Wandering

by Brenda Hooper

Lost and restless - how can we help them feel they belong?
Other people's reactions • Look for a pattern • Stay calm, distract,
don't confront • Safety and the "open door" approach • Good
building design and a welcoming atmosphere

Have you ever lost your car in a multi-storey car park? I remember an occasion when I did so. With increasing desperation, and fighting a rising sense of panic, I wandered up and down the lines of cars. People passed me, walking briskly and confidently straight to their cars. Only I, it seemed, was lost.

I forced myself to try and think logically, to recall at which end of the car park I had come in, and which arrows I had followed. But my wanderings had made me completely disorienated. I had lost all sense of direction.

Suddenly, right in front of me, there it was. Oh the relief! I was back in the land of those who knew where they were and where they were going. I almost fell into the driving seat, shaking with the fright I had had.

Feeling lost

But many elderly mentally infirm people stay lost. They never "find the car" but remain disorientated in a world of people who know where they are going. We may have occasional glimpses, like I did in the car park, of what it feels like to be lost, but to live permanently in surroundings that seem strange and unfamiliar is not something that most of us have to experience.

I remember a lady, in the early stages of dementia, standing near the window of her own sitting room, and saying in a bewildered voice "I don't recognise those curtains". She would sometimes, too, tearfully ask her daughter to take her home. She had never left her home but, spasmodically at first, and finally permanently, she no longer recognised it as her home.

Restless

Not all residents who wander are necessarily experiencing an acute sense of being lost. Physical restlessness does often, though, seem closely linked with mental restlessness. Most of us have experienced in ourselves an inability to sit still when we are waiting for an important phone call or for the postman to bring us a long awaited letter.

A demented person is unable to articulate why she is restless, but her behaviour demonstrates that she is disorientated and "feels" lost even when she is in her own home or in a very familiar environment.

Wandering can be an expression of the feeling of not knowing where she is, what is going on or what is about to happen. Being surrounded by people who clearly do know where they are going, and are moving briskly about their business, can add to the bewilderment and anxiety that the demented person feels.

How then can we help such people to

recapture the sense of belonging in a familiar environment, which we take for granted and which gives us our sense of identity?

Reactions

Some elderly people who wander may be obviously distressed or agitated. Others seem calm in themselves as they pace or potter around the room, and are sometimes described as "happy wanderers". However, these people can cause those around them, whether staff or other residents, to be anything but happy! It can be very frustrating to a busy carer to have to watch apparently aimless and constant restlessness and to feel unable to do anything about it.

The way other, mentally alert residents react may be one of the main problems. They may become irritated, impatient or distressed by the behaviour of the constant wanderer. It is a particular hazard if someone goes into other residents' rooms and disturbs or removes personal items. Most if not all elderly people will find it difficult to distinguish between this purposeless moving of objects and deliberate stealing. Frequent accusations of theft on top of the usual trail of mislaid items can seem just too much for hard pressed staff. It is even worse if the wanderer tries to get into someone else's bed!

This raises the issue of whether it is right to care for dementing people who display unsocial behaviour in the same setting as mentally alert elderly people. There are no easy answers in the integration/segregation debate. I believe there is a place for the specialist home or unit for extremely demented people whose behaviour is socially very unacceptable. But I also believe that a considerable degree of dementing behaviour can be managed in an integrated situation, and that sometimes other residents prove to be more tolerant and accepting than we might anticipate.

Observe

We must recognise, then, that wandering behaviour by residents is frequently a considerable problem for staff, but that there are approaches which can help in its management. In learning how to cope with a resident who wanders, the first essential is to make a careful observation of the behaviour and any patterns there may be in its occurrence.

This will lead on to a consideration of whether there are any discernable reasons for the wandering. Have we any idea why the resident wanders or why she wanders at the times she does? To answer these questions it is necessary to have some knowledge of the background and history of the person concerned. The procedures which are employed in order to manage the behaviour, will of course also be influenced by the physical characteristics and location of the home or hospital.

Familiarity in their environment provides reassurance to demented people even if they have lost the capacity to know where they are or to remember with whom they live. In a particular home a group of residents had to move to a new building. During the first few weeks one lady wandered a great deal more than she used to in the old building. It was clear that she did not yet recognise it as her home.

With the passage of time, she wandered less; she had clearly come to feel her surroundings to be more familiar. To help this forward, she had needed lots of reassurance, more staff contact than usual, and her attention directed to her own familiar belongings in her room.

Our sense of belonging in a familiar environment is linked with our own sense of personal identity, so anything that can be done to reinforce that self identification, can only help someone to be more at peace in her environment.

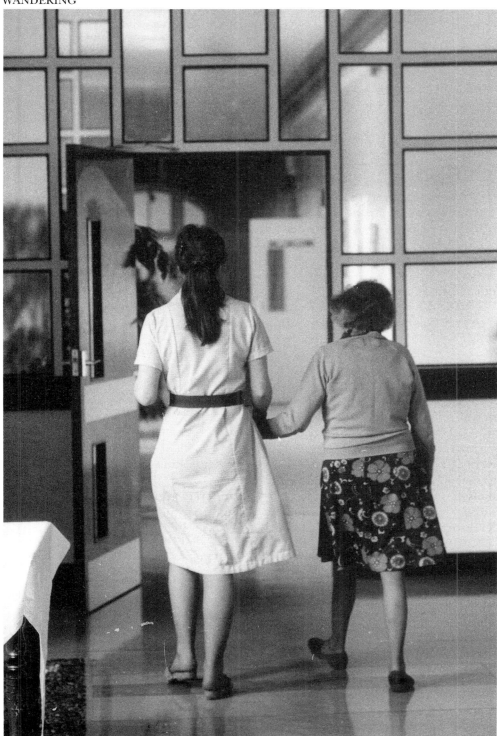

A short stroll, with some everyday conversation, may meet their immediate need.

Patterns

Wandering may look aimless, and some is, but in certain cases it may be possible to detect a pattern. Does the wandering happen mainly at night, or at a particular time of day, or does it seem to be triggered by some particular event? Beware of too quickly dismissing behaviour as being totally irrational. Perhaps it is possible to imagine how the person is seeing herself at the particular moment.

Is she an anxious mother, hurrying to pick up her children from school? Does she think it is Sunday and she is going to church? One resident always tried to go out at five o'clock in the evening, the time he used to take the dog for a walk.

A patient on a geriatric assessment ward would go into the garden, and then come back and pass urine in the ward. This was because he had lived all his life in a house with an outside lavatory – he had gone out to look for it. In one home, a particular lady was frequently found coming downstairs with her hat and coat on. Staff were frightened that she was about to try and leave the building. What it actually meant was that she had mistaken the day when her daughter was coming to take her out.

Action

How then can we use the information we gain about patterns of wandering and whatever understanding we have gleaned about the reasons for this? Calmness, reassurance, and lots of staff contact are essential. It may be difficult to treat an apparently irrational wanderer as a person with whom one can talk normally and rationally about the everday affairs of the home, but to do so may help as nothing else can, to bring her in touch at that moment with the world about her.

A golden rule is to distract, not con-front. Providing a cup of tea; a member of staff sitting down for a few minutes to have a chat or to look at some pictures together, may have a calming influence, at least for a while. If the person seems determined to go outside, then to go with her for a short stroll round the garden with some every-day conversation, may well meet the immediate need.

As we have seen, a detailed knowledge ot the person's background and previous lifestyle can help. If someone feels the need at five o'clock to go home and pre-pare the family's tea, then let them help with setting tables, filling milk jugs etc, for the residents' evening meal.

We must not forget the simple fact that some wandering may mean that the resident needs more physical exercise, or is bored!

Being able to go out for regular walks, and being involved with staff in simple activities for as much of the day as possible may help enormously. One very demented man enjoys helping the person who does the laundry to fold sheets. In one home, staff unexpectedly discovered the soothing effect on one of the residents of helping with planting out flowers; they had not previously known that she used to like gardening.

Remember above all, that in talking to demented people, tone of voice may be far more significant than the actual words used. If your own irritation or agitation is conveyed to the wanderer, this will only make things worse. A calm, friendly, soothing tone will be much more likely to achieve the desired result.

Most carers naturally pride themselves on their patience and understanding. However we are all human, and there will be occasions when we fail to act and speak in as controlled a way as we should. To recognise in ourselves the times when we are at our most vulnerable, and perhaps on occasions to ask another member of staff to help, is nothing to be ashamed of.

We can learn from one another how best to handle particular residents; and sometimes we just have to recognise that, through no fault of our own, a certain person responds better to another member of staff than to us. There may simply be something about a staff member that unconsciously reminds the resident of a much loved, or much hated relative.

Physical contact and the way we use it is as important as speech. The hand on the arm, or the arm around the shoulder, must convey a gentle desire to lead and to go along with, rather than a forceful pulling against, which will only be counterproductive.

If a resident seems anxious to leave the building, a reasonable suggestion to postpone going outside may sometimes be effective: "There will be a cup of tea soon – why not have that before you go out?". Of course, this does not always work.

One lady started wandering out very soon after she came to live in a certain home. At first staff tried straightforwardly to discourage her from going. This merely had the effect of making her aggressive and resentful. The house was large with several exits and a large garden, and she was clever enough to choose her moment and slip out (often inadequately clothed) by a back way while staff were busy elsewhere.

After this had happened a few times, and staff discovered to their surprise that amazingly she was able to find her way to her daughter's house, sometimes going on a bus, it was decided to pursue a different approach. Staff tried to be more understanding about her desire to go out (it was partly a response to a family who she felt neglected her). Sometimes they would use the diversionary tactic of a cup of tea, and this often worked. If it failed, they ensured that she had on a warm coat and proper shoes, and that her bus pass was in her handbag. Sometimes she then decided of her own accord that she wouldn't go out after all! Of course her family were also encouraged to visit her more regularly.

Open doors

What has been discussed above implies the acceptance of an open front (and back!) door policy. Many people doubt whether this approach can be justified when caring for vulnerable elderly people who are confused, or mildly or severely demented. Staff are understandably anxious about potential risk to the elderly person, and also concerned in case they themselves should be accused by relatives or other people of acting without due care and responsibility.

These are difficult issues. We must remember though, that an elderly person in care is entitled to the same basic rights as other people. This includes the right to liberty. Elderly mentally frail residents are not normally subject to the compulsory care or treatment provisions of the Mental Health Act, which involves medical intervention. Carers therefore have **no legal right to limit freedom**, and to restrain a resident could be considered an assault. There are certain circumstances where it may be permissible for someone to be physically restrained; for example if it is in self defence, to prevent a breach of the peace, or a crime, or when the consent of the person concerned can be implied or inferred. However, any such action would have to be able to be justified in law.

The crux of the matter lies in defining the professional responsibility of carers for the protection and safety of "wanderers" and how this should be interpreted in practice. We need to be very careful about assuming that our responsibility to protect a resident from physical harm outweighs the resident's right to freedom to come and to go at will.

There are, however, a number of strategies that can be adopted to reduce the likelihood of residents wandering out in circumstances which endanger their safety. There will be certain doors which it will be best to keep locked, but we must remember the vital necessity of keeping fire exit doors easy to open.

The front door may be tackled in various ways. It can be fitted with a handle that is too complicated for the demented resident to manage. The handle can be fixed low down, where she would be unlikely to find it. The door may be disguised as a window, by covering it with a curtain. An alternative or additional strategy is to site the office so that it affords a clear view of the front door.

Which of these approaches is adopted will depend partly on the location of the home, and on its nearness to busy roads. However many homes for very demented residents do in fact operate an open door policy, and the staff of one such home commented that the worst consequence any of their residents had suffered was a severe case of sunburn!

Missing

There will inevitably be occasions when a resident does go missing, and every home should have an agreed and written policy for the procedure to be followed. This will vary according to the situation of the home and known patterns of any frequent wanderers. Cultivating friendly relationships with neighbours can mean the swift return of a wanderer who has been spotted in the vicinity.

Informing police in advance of people who are likely to be found in the area can be helpful, as can the practice in one home of keeping to hand a description of a "regular" so that only the details of the clothes he was wearing when last seen needs to be added to the form before handing it to the police. It can be helpful too if potential wanderers carry on their person their name and address; but of course the dementia usually means there is no guarantee that a card placed in a wallet or handbag will remain there. Because of this some form of identity bracelet may be one solution.

Staff should also carry identification cards if they are involved in following a demented resident and trying to persuade them to return. This could prevent the embarrassing experience of explaining oneself to a policemen when an apparently lucid resident is complaining that "this person is following me"!

The importance of communication with residents' relatives must be stressed. It is vital that they are made fully aware of the home's policy about restraint and wandering, and that an anxious son or daughter is helped to understand the reason for the policy.

Using aids

There are a number of electronic aids to identification and restraint now on the market. Their use remains highly controversial. Most are similar to the system shops use to prevent theft. A small tag is secured somewhere about a resident's person, and a "pedestal" is placed in any doorway by which they might attempt to leave the building.

When the resident passes the pedestal, her tag completes an electronic loop that activates an alarm system, so that staff can bring her back to safety. Those who like the system say it does away with obtrusive and constant surveillance by staff. Opponents protest that tagging is an infringement of personal dignity, and that its use sets a very dangerous precedent.

The use of "geriatric" chairs with clip on tables and other physical restraints to prevent confused people getting up and moving freely around the room can never be condoned. They are a denial of the resident's right to freedom and dignity, out of a mistaken sense of responsibility. Special chairs for severely handicapped people used, with their consent, to prevent them falling forward involuntarily, are a different matter. We must not pretend that these are not difficult and thorny issues.

The use of sedation is another such question. There are times when a resident's restlessness and wandering is causing her such distress and is proving so impossible to modify or manage, that some medication is necessary. This should only be considered when other remedies have failed.

Medication must of course only be given when prescribed by a doctor, and its use and effects must be carefully and regularly monitored. In particular, minimal use should be made of daytime sedation and it should not be enough to cause drowsiness. We need to be particularly vigilant when a dementia sufferer cannot give informed consent to a proposed treatment.

Building design

A home with sufficient space for residents to wander freely indoors without coming to any harm, makes management much easier than in a small, confined, cramped building. At the stage of design of the building or perhaps in the planning of major alterations or extensions, the requirements of safety and proper supervision must be balanced with avoiding restricted access to personal space, that is to residents' own rooms.

A plan which is sometimes used is the so-called race track design, which provides a circular passage around a central courtyard. This ensures that residents can wander safely both inside and out of doors without feeling unduly restricted.

Smaller and non purpose built homes may of course find it more difficult to provide such a suitable layout, but some approximation to these principles may be aimed at. If there are stairs, then these may be a particular source of danger, and a gate may be appropriate. The aim should be to give space which allows for restlessness without encouraging repetitive wandering, and this is not always easy to achieve.

Relationships

Let us end our consideration on a positive note. However demented an elderly person, however intractable her wandering, the most constructive approach will be anything that will help to reinforce her own **sense of personal identity**. This means establishing and strengthening her relationships as an individual with the staff member who are often her most meaningful and regulare contacts.

Wherever possible a programme of shared activity, simple everyday things like helping to wash up, to clear the tables, to go for walks, to listen to music, to feed the birds, can all help to give her life some structure, familiarity and meaning.

An open, warm and welcoming atmosphere in all parts of the home or unit, without strict demarcations between staff and resident territory, will be one which will provide mentally frail elderly people with the frequent and reassuring contact they so much need.

Points to remember

1. Physical restlessness is linked with mental restlessness, with feeling lost and not belonging.

2. Recent change of surroundings, lack of exercise, boredom, can make wandering worse.

3. Look for patterns, times of day, what triggers it. Try to understand the reasons.

4. Distract, don't confront. Provide simple things to do, with staff.

5. Tone of voice is more important than words used. Be calm and reassuring.

6. Residents have a right to freedom. Physical restraint should rarely be used. Electronic methods are controversial.

7. Day time sedation should only be a last resort, and should not be used if it causes drowsiness.

8. Prepare for what to do when a resident goes missing.

9. An open door approach can work.

10. Be positive. Create a warm friendly atmosphere and good relationships with staff.

CHAPTER 8

Promoting hygiene and continence

by Ruth Manley

Hygiene as a daily routine • Bathing, showering, shaving,
hair care • Washing in bed or chair • Encouraging continence
• Managing incontinence of urine or faeces • Skin care

From childhood, the practice of keeping yourself clean forms an important part of everyone's daily routine. Washing or bathing, cleaning teeth, or washing hands before eating and after visiting the toilet, are regular features of everyone's day. These habits are important to people suffering from memory loss, as they can provide familiar activities at regular intervals. A normal routine like this helps confused people keep in touch with reality, occupies their time and gives reassurance. A hygiene care programme is also a useful framework for personal contact between individual staff and residents, and of course it helps to promote acceptable social behaviour.

The challenge to carers is to design regular routines which are supportive and helpful to residents, not staff. Routines should ensure that each resident receives the level of care required, but they must be flexible and give as much freedom of choice as each person can exercise. Too often regimes are restrictive with little regard for individual abilities. They seem designed for management or staff convenience rather than the wellbeing of each person.

Each member of staff should be encouraged to discuss specific goals for residents' hygiene programmes, and think about how these goals may be achieved.

Consider how difficult the problem becomes when a person is moved into a strange environment with different routines and no familiar face, and they suffer from mild to severe memory failure and anxiety. Elderly mentally infirm people are very afraid and insecure inside themselves. Looking after them is not easy, it is both challenging and time consuming.

So it helps if you can understand that residents are not being deliberately unco-operative when they resist regular washing or bathing. Standards and behaviour have changed a great deal during their lifetime; modesty was more prized in the past and today's frank body exposure causes distress to those unused to it. These old people can appear to us to be trapped in a time warp, clinging to what seem to be outdated conditions and behaviour unimaginable to young staff caring for them.

Staff must also come to terms with the different levels of psychological damage. Some residents may still retain a good standard of social conduct, needing only a little support. Others have some awareness and insight into what they are doing and what is happening to them, but they have significant memory loss and may become frightened or aggressive. Those whose dementia is severe, on the other hand, may become very benign and calm because they are blissfully unaware of much that goes on around them. They are extremely vulnerable and must be protected.

Cleanliness is important to both personal wellbeing and social acceptability, but as a consequence of ageing many people are unable to maintain the same standard of hygiene or grooming they previously enjoyed.

In their own home they may have been unable to heat or maintain the house properly, for example. Those in care may be affected by:

- Loss of energy or mobility
- Impaired sight or hearing.

Many elderly people also suffer from the effects or complications of a number of common conditions such as:

- Limb weakness following a stroke
- Partial loss of limb function after a bone fracture
- Breathlessness associated with chest or heart conditions
- Obesity
- Painful joints leading to reluctance to move
- Diseases affecting balance and coordination
- Blindness which restricts free movement
- Deafness which can reduce the ability to communicate or cooperate, and cause depression and isolation
- Incontinence as a result of underlying disorders.

What is your goal?

Here are some suggestions of what your aim should be for each resident:
1. To maximise a feeling of freshness and comfort.
2. To help the resident retain an interest in their appearance and standard of grooming.
3. To look after the skin and prevent damage to it.
4. To identify early signs of injury, rashes, or skin dryness or soreness.
5. To use the bathing/washing period to assess individual progress, such as change of mood, or ability to cooperate.
6. To note any physical signs such as pain on movement or "guarding" of a limb (reluctance to move it) for example, which may indicate injury or disease. This is especially important because severely confused people are unable to recall a fall or knock, or to report it.

How to achieve it

Weekly or more frequently as the condition permits:

Bath or shower in the bathroom. A bath may be more familiar for today's generation of old people, but showers are now standard equipment in many homes and younger residents may accept them without question. Remember that a warm bath is relaxing only if the bathroom is comfortably warm, draught free, and private.

Always work methodically. Plan the procedure logically along the following lines:
1. Prepare the environment. Close bathroom windows. Check the temperature of the room and water. Make sure before filling it that the bath is clean.
2. Collect towels, soap, flannels, and clean clothing together with any special items such as incontinence aids, lotions, creams or dressings.
3. Prepare the person. Remind them that it is their bathtime. Offer the opportunity to use the toilet. The sound of running water often makes people feel they want to pass urine. Wash the face in the handbasin before the bath, never in the bath. This is especially

important if the person is incontinent. Think how you would feel about having your face washed in water containing urine or faeces.

It is not a good idea to wash hair in the bath. Unless it is washed daily, hair becomes greasy and this grease combined with the shampoo prevents soap from lathering properly and cleaning skin effectively. Some shampoos may irritate sore or dry skin, causing itching.

Take great care when using a special bath, for example one which tilts, or a bath hoist. It is important for staff to fully understand and follow the manufacturer's instructions to ensure safety. These aids are useful for physically disabled or handicapped people who find movement painful or difficult. But some confused residents who cannot understand how the equipment works become very frightened and anxious, even aggressive and abusive. In the bath, let each individual wash as much of themselves as they can manage or be persuaded to do, assisting only when necessary.

Following the bath or shower the skin should be dried quickly and thoroughly. Talcum powder should be used sparingly, if at all; remember talcum powder is no substitute for adequate drying. When drying the feet inspect the toes and nails for redness, soreness, or moist patches between the toes which may indicate a fungal infection.

Check areas where skin surfaces are in contact, for example between the legs, under the breasts, or the cleft of the buttocks in obese people. Look for signs of soreness especially in hot weather when sweating is common. Report any skin areas which are red, cold and pale, or bruised. All abrasions and rashes must be examined by a senior member of staff.

Help the resident to dress, assisting them to do what they can, but not doing it all for them. Left to themselves it is likely that they will confuse the order in which garments are worn, but it is simple to observe and correct this while tidying the bathroom. Ensure that finger nails are clean and short, hair brushed or combed, and teeth cleaned.

Elderly people find a bath tiring so give them an opportunity to rest afterwards. Some residents prefer to have a bath during the evening so that they can put on their nightclothes, but this should not be encouraged if the bath is taken during the afternoon, nor must it become part of the day's routine to bath residents after lunch and then prepare them for bed. Remember that the aim of caring programmes for this group of elderly people is to maintain normality, and normal adults do not put on their night clothes in the middle of the afternoon.

Daily care

Each resident should be encouraged to wash their face and hands every morning and evening or be assisted by staff to do so. Washing the genital area of a continent resident is best carried out in the bathroom after visiting the toilet, using a disposable wipe. This may be a difficult procedure, however, if the person is suspicious or aggressive. A calm and persuasive manner is usually more successful at gaining cooperation, than confrontation. Diverting the attention by talking quietly combined with gentle handling is often successful in reassuring anxious or frightened people.

Finger nails are checked as part of daily hygiene routines. Give extra care to the nails of people with faecal incontinence to ensure cleanliness and prevent contamination. Volunteers sometimes offer regular manicures to residents, or staff take on this task as part of the home's activities.

Professional hairdressing may be provided on a regular basis, otherwise staff are responsible for hair washing. Washing every second week is adequate for most people, but those who smear as a result of incontinence, or have very greasy hair, need their hair washed as often as necessary.

Shaving

Most men are accustomed to shaving daily, and this is to be encouraged as a means of emphasising normal behaviour and good grooming. Help each man to retain his previous habits by allowing him to use his own razor and familiar method of shaving.

An electric razor is relatively safe and easy to use, provided the skin area being shaved is held taut while the razor head is rotated firmly across the bristles. It is important to unplug the razor and clean the heads after use before putting away. To prevent the spread of skin infection, never share a razor among a number of men. Wash and dry the face or wipe with a disposable wipe after shaving.

If the "wet" method of shaving is preferred, a safety razor is usually used. Shaving soap or cream is first applied to the beard with a brush or the fingers, and worked to form a lather. The razor is held at an angle to the skin which is held taut with one hand, and drawn with smooth strokes against the direction of bristle growth, removing hair and lather together.

To prevent scrapes or nicks of the skin it is important to hold the skin area being shaved firmly and to make clean strokes with the blade. Remaining lather is removed by washing and the skin dried. Dismantle the razor and discard the blade safely.

A number of elderly women suffer from facial hair and some have been accustomed to shaving to remove this. However this eventually leads to stubble, and the need to shave at very short intervals is a disadvantage.

An effective method for dealing with medium growth hair is the use of a depilatory cream applied in accordance with the maker's instructions. This gives a longer period of freedom from re-growth and is often more acceptable to the individual. These creams must not be used on sore or broken skin.

Whatever method of treatment is used it must be carried out in privacy. The practice of shaving women's superfluous hair in a public room is very insensitive.

Washing in bed or chair

Many residents are washed daily in their own rooms, either at a fitted handbasin or using a bowl at the bedside. Preparation for a strip wash is the same as for bathing in the bathroom: privacy, room temperature, and collection of equipment. People who can wash themselves will find it more comfortable to sit on the edge of the bed or in a chair with the bowl near at hand. Check that the water is comfortably hot and change it when it cools.

The feet are immersed in a bowl placed on a towel on the floor, soaking them to soften the nails if they are to be cut. Most older people need help to wash their back and feet, as they have difficulty in stooping.

Frailer or more severely confused residents may need to be washed completely by staff. In this case it is necessary to assess the best way of achieving maximum comfort with minimum disturbance in order to gain cooperation. This may mean you decide to wash the individual in bed.

Bedclothes must be removed before commencing the procedure, leaving the top sheet to cover the resident. It is advisable to have the water hotter when staff are washing someone because it loses heat quickly on the flannel, and feels cold to the skin. The water should be changed frequently and always after washing the genital area. The sequence of washing the body is usually "from top to toe" but this rule may be modified to meet individual needs.

Take great care when washing the "private parts", as many older people refer to the genital organs; some elderly ladies are very suspicious or modest about exposing this part of themselves. Nevertheless, to promote cleanliness and freedom from odour the vulval and anal areas must be gently sponged to remove secretions, with special care given to the skin folds of the groin and lips of the vulva. Always wash towards the anal opening so as not to contaminate the entrance to the bladder at the front.

The foreskin of uncircumcised men must be retracted in order to remove the debris which collects around the end of the penis. Exercise care in handling the penis and scrotum because these are very sensitive areas which become sore if handled carelessly. Thorough drying prevents soreness or chafing. A light dusting of talcum powder may be used, but too much produces caking.

Washing hair

Hair shampooing is best performed over a handbasin of adequate height or a basin on a table. Warm towels, a waterproof shoulder cape, jug of warm water for rinsing and shampoo which does not sting the eyes, brush and comb and hair dryer are collected. If a proper basin is available which permits the head to be tilted backwards this makes the task easier. You can also maintain eye contact which is reassuring for both of you. If not, warn the resident to close their eyes and hold their head over the bowl.

The hair is wetted, shampoo applied and massaged into the scalp. This is rinsed off and the process repeated. Rinse thoroughly until all trace of shampoo is removed. Wrap the hair in a warm towel and dry any splashes on the face or the ears. Remove excess moisture from the hair, then brush and comb, arranging in an appropriate style with a hand dryer.

Continence problems

Urinary or faecal incontinence increase the management problems for home staff in a number of ways, such as:
1. The protection of the environment, odour control, damage to carpets and furniture.
2. The protection of bedding and clothing.
3. The protection of residents' skin.
4. The disposal of soiled pads and pants.
5. The cost of laundry and replacement of linen.
6. Cost of labour and water heating.

All problems can be lessened or avoided by the introduction of toileting regimes, combined with a high standard of personal hygiene. Practical ways of promoting continence have been developed over the past fifteen years based on work undertaken by the Association of Continence Nurse Advisers. These plans of action are always based an individual's own pattern of going to the toilet, and they can be adapted with the help of the local nurse adviser to suit almost any group of clients. Specialist nurse advisers are based at your health authority, and you should be able to call on them for help. Manufacturers have developed a wide range of body worn aids and bed protection.

It is a mistake to assume that incontinence is an inevitable consequence of memory loss. Many people retain control of bladder and bowel in spite of advanced brain failure. Incontinence of recent onset must always be investigated by a doctor or experienced nurse, whatever the person's age or level of mental impairment. Urinary tract infection is very common: it has the effect of increasing confusion which improves once the infection is treated. If staff feel someone's incontinence problem should be investigated at a specialist clinic, your nurse adviser can help a great deal. Sometimes, however, investigation reveals no underlying treatable cause, and then the term intractable incontinence is used.

Incontinence of urine

The most important ingredient for sucess in carrying out toileting regimes is staff motivation and commitment. No continence programme can succeed without adequate staff training; the continence (nurse) adviser offers an invaluable advisory and educational role in the preparation of staff and assessment of residents. Unrealistic goals destroy the confidence of staff, who need much support during the early stages of all new programmes.

Individual assessment may include answering the following questions:

1. Can we identify any underlying cause?
2. How often is urine passed?
3. How much is passed each time?
4. How long has the person had a problem?
5. How aware are they of the incontinence?
6. How much cooperation are we likely to achieve?

In order to make assessment easier, staff may be asked to complete charts which show individual habits of passing urine over a period of days and nights. The resident is taken to the toilet at two or three hourly intervals, and the time and whether urine is passed or the person is wet is noted on the chart. If the amount of urine is to be recorded this is measured, or estimated if incontinence has already occurred.

Even when the resident is wet they should be taken to the toilet, to remind them that the toilet is the correct place for passing urine, and encourage complete bladder emptying. (Otherwise urine left in the bladder can become infected).

Habit training

The chart is used to see whether there is a pattern of passing urine. When the pattern shows that urine is passed at about the same time each day or night, staff plan a toileting regime which anticipates bladder emptying by taking the resident to the toilet around 15-30 minutes before the person is usually incontinent. This method is often very successful, but it cannot be used for someone whose pattern is erratic, as often happens in severely mentally impaired older people.

Set interval toileting

This regime involves reminding or taking the resident to the toilet at regular intervals. It is successful largely among people with memory loss who respond to staff intervention. It does not take individual habits into account, depending instead on regular toileting to prevent wetting. Set interval toileting is widely used in long stay institutions and by some older people living at home when memory failure or bladder awareness is lost.

Whatever regime is adopted it should not be rigidly imposed on every resident, because many confused people remain continent as long as there are adequate toilet facilities which are clearly signposted and marked, and as long as they are physically able to reach the toilet, with staff help if necessary.

Nevertheless there are some severely confused people for whom incontinence is inevitable. In order to preserve maximum dignity and comfort for this group, disposable pads and pants offer the best solution.

The great variety and quality of aids means professional assessment is needed to select the most suitable product for the individual. This assessment takes account of frequency and volume of urine, ease of use of the product, and disposability.

Skin care

The aim of skin care is to prevent soreness or skin breakdown by minimising contamination of the skin by urine. Many incontinence pads are designed to allow urine to pass through the inner layers to absorbent material underneath, away from the skin. Using catheters or sheaths to protect the skin from urine is not an option with confused people, who will try to remove them and may injure themselves.

Regular washing of the genital area is crucial to prevent smell and skin breakdown. But soap and water removes natural skin oils, so apply a cream afterwards to prevent excessive dryness or chafing. A barrier cream may be used to form a protective seal on the skin.

The risk of infection is high, because the combination of moisture, warmth, and contamination encourages bacterial growth. The risk is increased when there is faecal incontinence, and it is essential that staff do not further contaminate skin when cleansing the genital area after an episode of soiling. Disposable wipes are usually used because they make thorough cleansing easier, and so reduce infection and odour. Thorough drying is essential to protect skin.

Efficient disposal of soiled material such as pads, pants, or wipes helps to minimise unpleasant odour and cross infection. All soiled material must be handled carefully using disposable gloves, and placed in sealed bags for transport within the home or to the laundry. Adequate facilities for dealing with heavily soiled linen before laundering, and arrangements with local authority services for collection of contaminated material for incineration, are management responsibilities.

Incontinence of faeces

Episodes of soiling are fortunately less frequent than urinary incontinence. Diarrhoea or continual soiling must always be investigated and treated. A common cause of soiling is constipation, when liquid faeces leaks round a hard plug of solid faeces in the bowel. This "faecal impac-

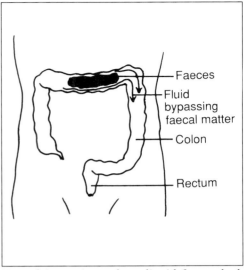

Faecal impaction, where liquid faeces leak around a solid plug of faeces in the bowel.

tion" is treated by a regime of dietery, drug, or other stool softening agents. Confused people may resist the use of enemas; and suppositories may be more acceptable. This treatment of faecal impaction may take several days or weeks if the constipation is long standing.

With age the anal muscles may become lax, cleansing following defaecation is more difficult and soiling occurs. The use of a damp wipe to complete the cleaning process may prevent this.

Care is aimed at protecting the skin from the effects of contamination. Skin breakdown inevitably leads to infection and pressure sores which are difficult to heal. In some very frail people they may even be fatal.

Staff should be alert to the possibility of confused people using inappropriate receptacles as toilet substitutes: litter bins, buckets, and handbasins for example remind residents of the toilet and may be so used.

Sometimes unpleasant surprises face staff. One resident hid faecal matter in her handbag, under the pillow or mattress, and in her jewel box. She obviously knew that her behaviour was inappropriate and made great efforts to conceal the faecal matter. This resident did not recognise herself in a mirror, could not recognise a toilet, and did not know her son.

Someone suffering from brain failure is very vulnerable and dependent upon the kindness and tolerance of others. Neglect of appearance and failure to maintain normal standards of cleanliness is often what has brought about the admission into care. All staff have responsibility for maintaining acceptable hygiene standards, but management policy, training and supervision of staff, are crucial. Management aims must be clearly defined and achievable, based on supporting both residents and staff in what is often a frustrating and challenging environment.

Points to remember

1. Remember that residents have differing levels of mental function and confusion. This affects goal setting in the development of hygiene regimes. The aim is to encourage each person to continue normal standards of cleanliness.

2. Consider the factors which prevent residents from maintaining acceptable hygiene standards. Set goals which are based on individual need. Use hygiene programmes to provide general well-being and staff/resident contact.

3. Recognise that incontinence is not an inevitable consequence of brain failure. Utilise the support and experience of the Continence Nurse Adviser in promotion of continence programmes. Consider how toileting regimes can be introduced for individual residents.

4. Develop strategies to reduce skin damage resulting from urinary or faecal incontinence. Remember that the combination of moisture, warmth, and contamination increases the risk of pressure sores. Prevent cross infection and unpleasant odour by adopting safe methods of waste disposal.

5. Accept that ultimate responsibility for severely impaired old people lies with individual staff members.

CHAPTER 9

Eating and drinking

by Pauline Crawford

Thinking on behalf of your residents • Nutritional needs • Mealtimes as social occasions • Help with feeding • Importance of fluid and fibre in the diet

The elderly person you are caring for may not know the correct time of day, day of the week, the month or year. Eating is a habit and social activity as well as a biological need, so you can see that a confused state of mind may well result in altered appetites. The person may have little appetite and inclination to eat; or on the other hand have a desire to eat often, sometimes inappropriate food or even non-edible items. Clearly, they are not thinking about what they ought to eat. They need you to pay attention to food and drink for them.

Nutritional needs

People generally require fewer calories as they grow older. Metabolism, or the rate at which the body uses up calories, slows down with age. However, if the mentally infirm person is very active, they could require as many calories as a younger person. Their weight should be monitored regularly.

A balanced diet consists of protein, vitamins, carbohydrates, minerals, fibre and fats. Protein is needed to maintain healthy tissues and prevent muscle wasting. Fluid requirement is two litres per day. That is eight to ten cups of tea, water, juice or any fluid of choice.

Reminders

Confused people may forget either that they have just eaten or which meal is next; you may have to gently remind them. It helps to talk to residents about the meal that is being prepared. Discuss the menu – this may remind residents of meals they enjoy, and can evoke memories.

Meal times are an aid to orientation. What people say and do at meal times re-affirms the time of day and the behaviour associated with it. Special days, such as Christmas and Easter, can bring further aids to orientation, with decorations as well as special foods.

Music is always recognised by areas of the brain, and can affect behaviour. Lively music, not too loud, played just before meal times, can increase the appetite and enjoyment of food. Quieter, more melodic music can aid relaxation and rest if it is played following the meal.

Remember that a visit to the toilet before the meal starts, assures comfort for the resident and reduces disruption during the meal itself. Comfort is continued by another visit following eating and drinking. All these actions, with attention paid to personal hygiene, are part of the total care you give each resident.

Mealtimes are a recognised social occasion. The most natural position for eating is to sit upright at a table. In our society we like to share the occasions of meal times with others, family and/or friends. Should any resident have anti-social habits when eating, it is tactful to position them away from others who can maintain eating habits that we regard as "normal".

Feeding

Co-ordination in transferring food from the plate to the mouth can present a problem for some people. Also the muscles which govern chewing and swallowing may not be able to cope with some foods, and softer diet may be more appropriate. Dentures, if worn, should be clean and well fitting.

When using a knife, fork or spoon is a problem, special utensils with thicker handles may help. Sponge or rubber grips can be placed over handles. Look at the needs of each person individually. If retaining food on the plate is a problem, plate guards are very effective. A non-slip mat below the plate prevents it sliding on the table top.

Supervision is required during meals to monitor how each person is coping. Maintaining independence is always preferable if it can realistically be achieved. But food can become cold and unappetising, so a degree of help with feeding may be required.

Always sit alongside the person you are helping to feed. Offer small, easily managed mouthfuls. Keep foods separate so that individual flavours can be tasted and appreciated. Allow rest periods after each swallow.

Most of your residents will probably require smaller meals more often during the day. Finger shaped sandwiches of egg, cheese or meat, are very useful for snacks.

Consider how food is presented. The ageing process affects eyesight and the senses of taste and smell, which all become less efficient. How do you think a plate of chicken, creamed potatoes and cauliflower would look? Nutritionally very good but bland to say the least!

As you try to ensure an adequate fluid intake you may find that full cups of tea are not appreciated. During the day small amounts of fluids, offered often, are more readily accepted. Sips of fluid between mouthfuls of food help to assist swallowing, and rinse the mouth naturally. Drinks that are either very cold or very hot are not readily tolerated by elderly people. This does not mean that everything from tea to water should be of the same temperature, rather that if you want to encourage fluid intake you need to think about temperature.

Fruit juices, high in vitamin C, assist with nutrition. So do small pieces of fruit which are high in vitamin C, such as tangerines or oranges. A small piece of tinned pineapple contains enzymes which encourage the production of saliva and naturally clean the mouth.

Constipation

Food is digested in the stomach and small intestine, and when it enters the bowel, or colon, it is fluid. The main function of the bowel is to absorb water; this continues until the semi-solid consistency of faeces is attained. Mineral salts and some drugs are also absorbed by the colon.

In considering the overall effect that eating and drinking have on the wellbeing of your resident, let's have a look at what can often become a problem. The miseries of constipation for elderly people include loss of appetite, furred tongue, unpleasant breath and abdominal discomfort. This is particularly noticeable in a confused elderly resident who will already have changes in appetite. In addition constipation results in increased confusion and agitation; this is caused by increased gases in the blood stream affecting the brain.

When faeces become more solid in the bowel and cannot be helped along by the bowel's muscular action, faecal fluid may

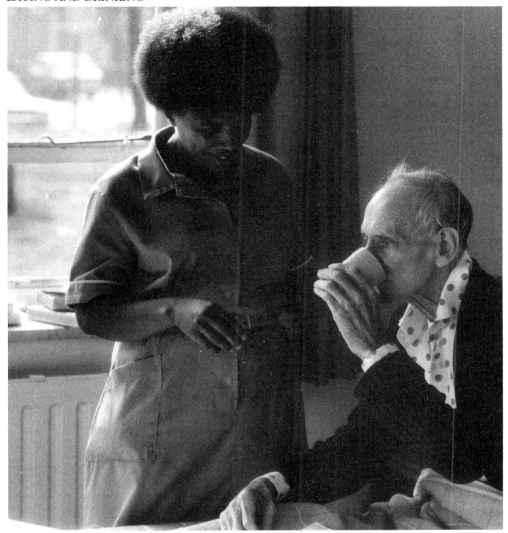

Small amounts of fluid, offered often, are more readily accepted than full cups.

by-pass the solid matter. This can be mistaken for diarrhoea.

The by-passing fluid could lead to incontinence in a previously continent person, or increase incidences of incontinence. It is important to recognise these signs and symptoms and report them correctly to your superior.

The causes of constipation are many. Firstly the muscular action of the bowel is slower and less efficient in elderly people. Fibre in the diet adds bulk to the faeces and assists movement of the bowel. Lack of adequate fibre reduces the bulk and does not stimulate bowel movement. Physical activity, moving and walking about, assists the muscles in the bowel. Reduced mobility therefore increases constipation in elderly people. Inadequate fluid intake will cause constipation. Especially in the warm environment of a care home, the body needs plenty of fluid, otherwise faeces will become hard and therefore increasingly difficult to move along the bowel.

Dehydration

Dehydration occurs when someone's fluid intake is really inadequate. The signs and symptoms are increased confusion, dry skin with loss of elasticity (when the skin is gently pulled to one side, it is very slow to return to its former position) dry mouth and tongue. A dry mouth and tongue not only prevents someone enjoying their food but also leaves the mouth open to infection.

Aside from problems with diet and fluids, there are drugs such as water tablets (diuretics) and some painkillers (analgesics) used for arthritis, which also cause constipation and dehydration.

There are further problems which arise from constipation and dehydration. Leakage of faecal fluid increases the risk of urinary tract infections especially in females. This is because the urethra, the tube from the bladder to the outside, is much shorter than in males, and bacteria can find a route into the bladder and cause infection. An infection will cause discomfort and increased urgency, which can result in increased incontinence.

Dehydration means the bladder is not being filled adequately, the natural stimulus to empty the bladder is absent, and waste products are not being flushed away in urine as nature intended. If urine is stagnant in the bladder the waste products break down and cause infection.

Your care

The mentally infirm elderly person is unable to comprehend the importance of a balanced, suitable diet. They rely totally on you, the carer. It is a very important part of the total care you offer to them. Their welfare and well-being is in your hands.

We have looked at the basic nutritional needs, some important actions in feeding and drinking, the possible complications which may occur and what they may mean to the individual concerned. Your challenge as carer is to fulfil your residents' nutritional and meal time social needs as far as you possibly can, by thinking and acting on their behalf.

Points to remember

1. You must think about food and drink on your residents' behalf.
2. Give information specifically, and often, to residents.
3. Think about the position they are in when eating and drinking.
4. Think about what they are eating and drinking.
5. Be aware of the complications arising from an unbalanced diet, especially constipation and dehydration.
6. Observe residents, and report any changes or symptoms of ill health.
7. Remember what an important job you are doing!

CHAPTER 10

Keeping people moving

by Stuart Darby

• The effects of normal ageing • How mental health affects mobility • Promoting independence • Lifting and handling • Using equipment

Mobility is the process in which muscles and joints work together to allow an individual to undertake some form of active movement. It is important because it allows each older person the opportunity of freedom and choice, to do what they want to, when they need or want to. It affords each one the dignity and privacy to be able to carry out movement and daily living activities without interference or intrusion. Finally it permits fulfilment and a sense of satisfaction in being able to cope with and control everyday tasks, preventing frustration and anxiety.

The older person may be a patient, resident, relative or tenant, but each one is a unique individual, and we need to ask the same questions to achieve the goals of mobility:

1. How can I assist this older person to be independent in caring for themselves?
2. What information and guidance can I provide to prevent them losing any mobility?
3. How can I ensure that the older person with limited mobility is moved safely and with dignity?

A knowledge of the physical and mental changes that can cause immobility helps to anticipate and prevent, as well as recognise, present problems in older people.

Physical changes in old age

These include normal "wear and tear" to the body, or part of the process of an illness or disease:

(a) Decreased elasticity of muscles and the inability to bend and flex easily.

(b) A decline in strength of bones (bones become thinner in older age).

(c) Reduced lung expansion causing breathlessness on exertion.

(d) Poor eyesight and inability to recognise objects, steps or floor changes; this increases the risk of falls and accidents.

(e) Changes in the inner ear may cause loss of balance control.

(f) Medicines and alcohol may act more potently with older people, causing drowsiness and unsteadiness.

(g) Heart changes, causing the blood pressure to rise or fall quickly, may make the old person dizzy or unsteady.

(h) Pain in the hands or limbs, caused by rheumatism or arthritis, can limit the full range of movement needed to stay active.

Mental health changes

Changes in mental health affect a small percentage of older people, influencing many aspects of their life and affecting mobility.

Memory and orientation

Remembering and recalling information such as where they are (the time, month or year), what is happening around them, or what they were doing, can create problems for the older person. It can lead to repeated questioning and searching for clues to make sense of, or keep in touch with the world around them. Wandering means that poor vision and lighting may place the older person at risk if walking alone.

Communication

Difficulty in finding the right words, making up words or stopping mid-sentence affects mobility if we are unable to understand what the older person is trying to convey. It is important to ensure that instructions for movement and activity are understood and able to be carried out by the older person. Making sense of what is going on, and what is seen or heard can help to allay frustration and aggression (reality orientation, described in chapter 3, is very useful here). Inappropriate reactions or behaviour may be displayed if the older person feels threatened or suspicious of the actions of others.

Behaviour

The main behaviour disorders that develop – wandering, noisiness, incontinence and "stripping-off" – have been dealt with in previous chapters. The older person acts in a way that they feel is appropriate, rational and logical. Conflict is caused if situations are not handled appropriately and diplomatically. It is important that any activity or mobility is not brought to a halt, but channelled into productive and useful movement. Wandering may be the opportunity to go for a walk, and stripping off, for example, a time to change clothes.

Control

Older people with mental illness have a tendancy to limit and restrict their environment in order to remain "in control" of it. Interests and activities may dwindle, or be forgotten. There may be resistance to active movement, where the older person is anxious and feels insecure about being unable to control the situation.

"Clinging" can occur where the older person has experienced a fall, and lost self confidence in mobilising. Reassurance, plenty of time and simple stages to approaching any activity of mobility are essential to overcome this.

Insight

There may be occasions when the older person is aware of, and tries to hold on to, periods of insight and reality. Personal possessions, individual walking sticks, frames and personal property will help them to maintain a sense of ownership and belonging.

Confusion

Confusional states may be temporary, as a result of alcohol, drugs, illness or disease, or permanent. Inability to recognise people, places or objects can create problems where, for example, the floor covering is mistaken for a step and obstacles and furniture are not seen or recognised.

Mood

The mood of the older person can fluctuate between extremes of being happy and relaxed, to being sad, anxious or agitated. Concentration on tasks, walking or carrying out movement, needs to be planned to take place in small appropriate stages. Feelings of uselessness, apathy or a recent bereavement will clearly affect motivation and continued activity. Positive encouragement, and ensuring a sense of satisfaction and achievement will help the older person to remain mobile.

Mobile and independent

Establishing a close relationship with the older person will enable you to observe, identify problems and contribute to the plan of care for mobility. Promoting independence, assessment and care plans, and the equipment that you use, are essential components.

Promoting independence

1. Movement or activity will be influenced and conditioned by the **past lifestyle, type of work, leisure activities, education** and **life experiences** that the older person may have had. Using past experiences as a guide to plan and encourage future activity that will be acceptable to the olde person, is likely to have a high degree of success.

2. The older person may have **different attitudes, values** and **beliefs** from younger people. They might not, for example, respond if the wrong name is used. Certain activities, for example cooking, may not appeal to older men, who may be unwilling or unmotivated to join in with an activity.

3. The **perception of the older person,** how they feel about you, the society or community around them, will influence how they respond and behave. We need to keep in mind cultural differences and expectations of the older person. One such example includes the use of shower equipment that is not "normal" to many older people. Velcro, used to fasten clothing, may be seen as unnatural, and the opening action perceived as ripping or tearing clothing. Keeping things as normal as possible for as long as possible is the key to maintaining a real world.

What are assessment and care plans?

It is usual for a qualified nurse, physiotherapist or occupational therapist to determine the long term approach to mobility for each individual. An assessment contained in a care plan should include the following features:

1. The **ability of the client to understand and contribute** to their own movement to ensure that independence is maintained, and the continued use of their muscles and limbs.

2. The **height and weight** of the client. This is important to ensure that you are aware of that weight and prepared to lift it.

3. Assessment of the patient's **physical abilities** includes:

• Use of one or more arms/legs.

• Ability to turn, sit or stand up.

• Ability to support some or all of their own weight.

• Ability to walk, and the distance, with or without equipment.

• Evidence of illness or disease.

• Side effects of medicine or alcohol that may be causing drowsiness or dizziness.

4. **The number of people required to assist.** Never try alone to lift or help an older person stand if you know that two or more people are required. The older person who is agitated, misunderstands your actions, or is unable to help, has special needs.

Equipment

Equipment such as special beds, chairs, hoists, sticks or frames must be carefully chosen and measured for individual use. A frame or stick that has been measured for one person, can only be safely used by that person. Hoists and mechanical aids will have specific instructions. Learn how to use this equipment, and follow any manufacturer's instructions.

Lifting and handling

Clothing and footwear

Uniforms should be designed to take into account the movements that you will need to make. They must allow you to bend and stretch freely. Where no uniform is worn, it is important that you select clothing that allows free movement, but is unlikely to be caught in equipment.

Rubber-soled shoes protect us from static electricity and are non-slip on wet or polished surfaces. The upper surface is also important to protect feet from articles or objects that may be dropped upon them, including the odd misplaced walking stick.

It is equally important for older people to wear well-fitting shoes that support the foot and ankle, and not loose fitting slippers. Remember also that long hair, rings and jewelry can get trapped in equipment.

Planning a lift

Being prepared involves knowing how to lift and move safely to protect:

• The safety of the older person

• Your own personal safety

• The safety of other staff, colleagues and visitors to the area in which you work.

Do I need any help to lift?

Ask questions or seek help if you are unsure or don't think that you can manage the lift. Only use procedures with which you are familiar. Do not guess the correct procedure or try to improvise when lifting or moving.

Is the area clear?

Make sure you have enough space in which to move around, and that the distance that you will be travelling is clear of objects and furniture. If you are transferring a person from one place to another, for example bed to chair, ensure that these are at the same level.

Plan your move to take into account the number of different stages: standing, turning, sitting and so on. Lower any handrails or chair sides to minimise the amount of lifting and lowering required. Be sure to lock the wheels of equipment, and position, for example, a chair or bed ladder which may help the older person to help themselves.

Is the floor safe?

There may be obstacles such as furniture or rugs and carpets. The floor may be wet, polished, covered in talcum powder or another slippery substance. Do remember that pets may also be a hazard that you need to look out for.

Preparing the person

Before starting to move or lift, the reasons for, and the purpose of the procedure need to be explained clearly and concisely. Take time to ensure that the older person understands what is going to happen. It may be necessary to use signs, gestures or other forms of communication to ensure that the older person is able to join in with any activity and is not alarmed by any procedure. Communication includes the words that are used, the tone and volume in which you speak as well as the pace at which you speak. Body language – the way we look at a person, how close we move towards them, and how we touch them – can be more important than words alone.

Consider the following steps:

Can I lift or do I need to lift?

Perhaps the older person could move himself given time and help. Allow yourself plenty of time to undertake this activity. Explain clearly:

WHY the older person should move.
WHERE you want the older person to move to.
WHAT you intend to do.
WHAT you want the older person to do to assist you or help themselves.
WHEN you are going to start the procedure.

PREPARING TO LIFT

Have I chosen the right grip and lift?
A planned procedure will take a limited amount of time, and cause less distress. Alternative methods and procedures may be recommended and adopted specifically for use in your own work situation.

Am I in the right position?
Position your feet to prevent twisting or bending your upper body. Face the direction in which you intend to move, with your chin tucked in, and focus your mind and

eyes completely on the activity.

Are my feet apart?

Correct foot positioning is essential to maintain balance. Keep your feet at least one hip breadth apart. Point one foot in the direction in which you will be moving; try to keep this foot slightly forward of the other if possible. Moving your feet instead of your body can help to maintain your balance and reduce the risk of strain on back and stomach muscles.

Is my back straight?

Imagine a piece of string attached to the top of your head, and tied to the ceiling (in a straight line but not necessarily vertical. This will help to keep your back straight, ensuring that any weight you lift is spread evenly through your body and that no pressure is placed in one particular area.

Are my knees bent?

Lower back muscles are not very strong. It is essential therefore that you use leg muscles to lift. By squatting down, bending at the knees, with the back straight (remember that piece of string), you can avoid strain on back muscles and lift more weight.

Is the load close to my body?

Holding the person close to your body will cut down on the amount of stress exerted on your arms and back. This can also reassure older people and help them to feel safer and more secure as you carry out the lift. But do remember that some older people may not like the close contact.

Is my grip firm?

The correct grip minimises the strain when lifting. Muscles can be stretched when not ready for action, or used quickly without thought. If you do not feel that you have a good grip you are likely to try and "hold-on" and consequently cause an injury to yourself.

Am I concentrating on what I'm doing?

All of these actions need to be part of a planned activity. Never rush or become complacent about helping older people to mobilise. This is frequently the time when accidents and injury occur. A knowledge and understanding of the principles for lifting is essential for safe movement.

Grips and grasps

There are a number of grips or grasps that you can safely use when helping older people to move, as well as "lift-up" seats that can be purchased. If the person may become agitated or physically aggressive remember to choose a grip that will also limit movement – *for the briefest time possible and only where they are unable to help themselves.* Keep your grip firm, but relaxed. Take care not to pinch or drag the skin.

After lifting

Always return furniture and fittings to their normal position. Place equipment or furniture in familiar places to decrease confusion

---

PREPARING TO LIFT

1. Am I concentrating?
2. Can I lift or do I need to lift?
3. Do I need any help to lift?
4. Is the area clear?
5. Is the floor safe?
6. Have I chosen the right grip and lift?
7. Am I in the right position?
8. Are my feet apart?
9. Is my back straight?
10. Are my knees bent?
11. Is the person held close to my body?
12. Is my grip firm?
13. Is my chin tucked in?
14. Am I lifting with my leg muscles?
15. Am I using gentle movements?
16. Am I likely to twist or bend?

The two-person lift - for transferring

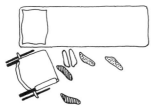

Correct position of wheelchair and helpers' feet

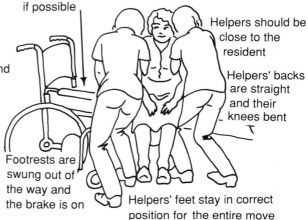

Arm of wheelchair should be removed if possible

Helpers should be close to the resident

Helpers' backs are straight and their knees bent

Footrests are swung out of the way and the brake is on

Helpers' feet stay in correct position for the entire move

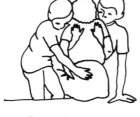

Back view

1. Starting position

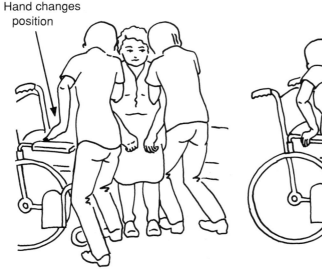

Hand changes position

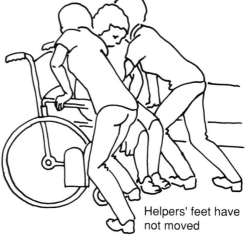

Helpers' feet have not moved

2. Help the resident clear of the bed

3. Turn and lower her into the wheelchair

The shoulder lift - for lifting up the bed

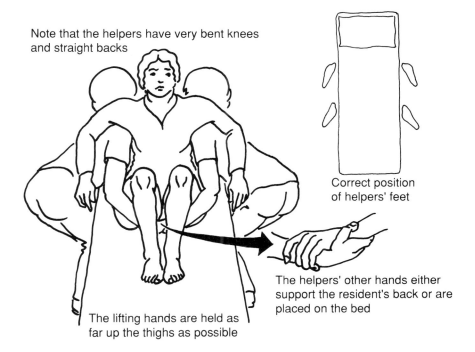

Note that the helpers have very bent knees and straight backs

Correct position of helpers' feet

The helpers' other hands either support the resident's back or are placed on the bed

The lifting hands are held as far up the thighs as possible

Moving from bed to chair   Through arm lift (two people)

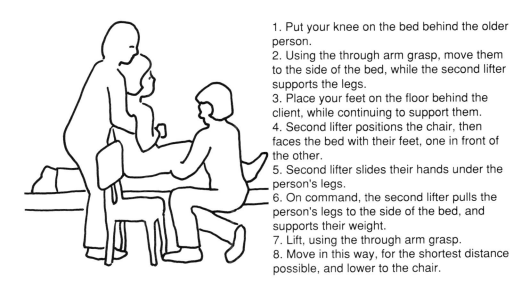

1. Put your knee on the bed behind the older person.
2. Using the through arm grasp, move them to the side of the bed, while the second lifter supports the legs.
3. Place your feet on the floor behind the client, while continuing to support them.
4. Second lifter positions the chair, then faces the bed with their feet, one in front of the other.
5. Second lifter slides their hands under the person's legs.
6. On command, the second lifter pulls the person's legs to the side of the bed, and supports their weight.
7. Lift, using the through arm grasp.
8. Move in this way, for the shortest distance possible, and lower to the chair.

Lifts for use by one person

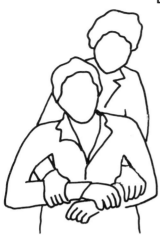

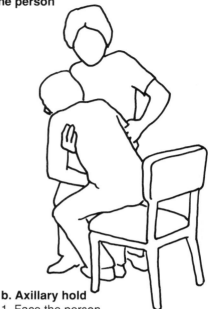

Helping the older person to stand:

a.Through arm grasp

1. Hold the person's forearm close to their body. If they have any weakness, their stronger hand should grasp their weaker wrist.
2. Stand directly behind them.
3. Grasp as near to their wrist as possible, and tuck their hands into the lower abdomen.
This lift can be used where the person is seated in an upright position and where they are able to stand, carry some of their own weight and can understand and cooperate.

b. Axillary hold

1. Face the person.
2. Place your leading foot beside the older person.
3. Place your other foot to block their feet and knees.
4. Place your other hands under their axillae(underarms).

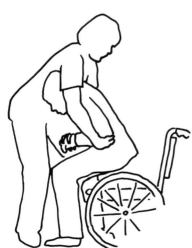

Assisting the older person from wheelchair to toilet

Elbow lift

1. Place the wheelchair in front of the toilet (brakes on).
2. Move the older person, using a side to side rocking movement, to the front of the chair.
3. Raise the footplates, and place their feet on the floor.
4. Loosen their clothing.
5. Stand directly in front of the older person, blocking their feet with your own feet.
6. The older person is asked to grasp their wrists together. You grasp their elbows, while leaning slightly forward and over.
7. The older person is rocked from front to back until they are standing.
8. Move them to one side, until your position and the position of the older person are exchanged.
9. Gently lower to the toilet.

and disorientation. Return equipment to its normal storage place for use by other people. If any equipment does not appear to be working properly, report it, and either remove or clearly label the faulty item.

Reporting back

Any changes observed in the older person, or any difficulties encountered, should be reported back to the person in charge as soon as possible. You may discover a positive way of helping somebody, or that they respond to a particular approach, that could help others when working with that person.

Conclusion

Mobility, the action of muscles and joints, is something that we all take for granted. For some people, the process of mobilising needs great determination and effort, particularly where physical and mental changes have taken place that reduce the full range of movements.

Promoting independence ensures that each individual can continue to live as independently as possible, permitting them to be fulfilled in maintaining their dignity and self esteem. When assisting the older person through lifting and handling, it is essential that their own abilities are encouraged, and that any movement is carried out with the safety of everyone in mind.

Points to remember

1. Mobility is important because it allows each older person the opportunity of independence, freedom and choice. It permits fulfilment and a sense of satisfaction in being able to cope with and control everyday tasks.

2. Each individual older person will undergo both physical and mental changes that affect their mobility. A knowledge and understanding of these changes can help to anticipate and prevent, as well as recognise present problems.

3. Promoting independence is an essential component of mobility. Establishing close working relationships, observing, identifying and contributing to plans of care for mobility will ensure that the older person remains independently active for as long as possible.

4. Assisting the older person to be independent is the main aim at all times. A knowledge of how to lift and move safely, is a key component to protect your own health, and the health of the older people with whom you work.

5. It is essential to report any changes in the older person's condition to the appropriate person in charge. It is equally important that any faulty equipment is clearly labelled, reported and removed from use.

CHAPTER 11

Relatives

by June Andrews

All relatives are different • Good reasons why their involvement is different • They will be anxious, and you can help • Good and bad ways of communicating • Responding to complaints • Relatives' support groups • Death in the family

When dealing with relatives it is important to remember a few key points:

• all relatives are different, so their involvement will be different

• relatives may be anxious, and you can help them by anticipating their fears

• if you welcome questions and help find answers it will make relatives less anxious

• you can ensure practical information is available to them

• the way you tell relatives about the care of your elderly residents can affect the way they feel

• complaints can be a good thing if they are handled sensitively

• relatives are often adjusting to a great change and you are very important in making that possible

• relatives often get support from each other

A large number of elderly people live at home alone. Some have living relatives; some do not. The amount of contact with those relatives varies.

Think about your own family. There may be some old relatives, for example an old aunt, that you send a card to at Christmas, but who lives too far away to visit. On the other hand, your grandma may live in the same town as you, and be visited each day by a stream of children and adults, so she actually has to get out of the house for a bit of peace and quiet. Then there may be an old uncle no one has heard of for years, and you sometimes wonder if he is still alive.

Individuals

The important thing to remember is that every old person is different, and their relatives are different. Some old couples only have each other, and if one of them becomes very frail, the other may have to arrange for a home, because they cannot cope any more.

Who is the relative?

The relative of your latest resident may be a husband or wife, son or daughter, nephew or niece, brother or sister, granddaugher or grandson. The relationship might be an informal one.

For example, the person who comes and takes most interest might be the man who has lived with your elderly resident for the last twenty years as her lodger. He means more to her than any of her cousins, and you may have as much contact with him as them.

What influences the way they are?

The way the relatives behave towards the

home and staff, and the elderly resident, depends on what their relationships have been like in the past.

• "Mum is in a home just three miles from us so we can call round in the car every day, and if the weather is nice, she comes out with us when we go to do the shopping and buys a few bits for herself. When everyone comes to our place for a party, we either fetch her along, or take the party to her, and her friends can see what a big crowd we are and join in the fun. We've almost 'adopted' the women at her place, and they know all of us".

• "I hadn't really spoken to my aunt since I was a child, but as I am a solicitor the family looked to me to make all the arrangements about the home and other financial details. Actually, my brother who is a nurse would have been a better choice. Anyway, they know at the home that they can write to me if there are any problems, but I don't see the point of asking to speak to her. She doesn't know who I am anyway."

With each of these relatives you can see what the position was before the change of coming into a home. This explains why some relatives have less contact.

How will they react to the home where you work?

The way people react is very different, but there are a few things you can guess.

If they have experience of what a home is like they will compare you and your surroundings with that. They may have looked at a number of places before choosing yours, so at least you know that you must have some good points. If they find other things that trouble them you may do a lot to make them less anxious. They may not ask you directly, but if you listen very carefully to what they say, you may be able to guess what is troubling them.

For example, a son might say, "It"s a long way to the dining room from the bedroom". You might think that he was complaining, and think that it is not his problem. You might say, "Yes and my feet are killing me by the end of the day!" But if you listen again you will hear that what he is really saying is "My dad can't really walk that far in the morning. Will he be all right?" Your answer could be to explain what you do to overcome the problem of the distance, by serving breakfast in bed, or having a buffet breakfast bar where people can get breakfast at any time up till lunch, no matter how slow they are at getting going in the mornings.

You are important

You can also predict that the relatives may be anxious. They may have gone through a great deal of trouble to make this arrangement and they are anxious that nothing should go wrong. When people are anxious they behave in strange ways. Have you ever been to an interview and found yourself laughing nervously at the wrong time and dropping things? Do you remember waiting for ages to see a doctor and then coming out unable to remember what he said, and with a list of unanswered questions in your head?

You might not think, if you are working as a care assistant in a residential or nursing home, that you make other people nervous, but you should consider the possibility. You are very important to relatives. What you seem to think and feel about their elderly relative can make all the difference between them feeling good or feeling bad about the whole place.

But of course it can work either way. Either the relatives hang on to your every word, and go home and worry about all that you said, or they ignore you and ask to see the person in charge. If you are always willing to talk, they will eventually discover that you are likely to be able to help or to find out information for them. A word from you about how the resident is doing, or a quote, can make the relative feel better.

•"Janice (she's the little care assistant, who works mornings) says that whenever dad wakes up he asks for me, and she tells him that I'll be along at the weekend. That keeps me going now. I used to get him up myself, every day, and now he doesn't even recognise me when I sit with him."

Janice is giving the daughter the thanks for all her years of care that she will never hear from the lips of her old confused father.

What kind of questions will they ask?

Relatives will often ask the kind of questions that will be answered by this book. Other questions include general information about your residential home that you can answer yourself. Some questions that they ask will seem to have no answer.

People might ask about:

• your residential home

• the care of the elderly person

• complaints

• other things that you have to make sure are passed on

Your home

There may be a leaflet that can be given away that will help the relatives to remember some of the information about your home. If there is not, you might be a good person to design it, as the person who does most of the personal care of the resident and therefore has a lot of contact with relatives. You know the kind of questions that can be asked.

Try to fill in this information form from memory, and then ask around to find out the extra information that you need.

NAME OF HOME

RESIDENT'S FULL POSTAL ADDRESS INCLUDING POST CODE

TELEPHONE NUMBER AND CODE

NAME OF THE PERSON IN CHARGE AND THEIR QUALIFICATIONS

LOCATION: How to get there (Maps, and details of public transport might help, and approximate cost of a taxi if necessary)

VISITING: The details of restrictions (if any) or an encouragement to open visiting. Where the visits may take place: in the residents room, or a private sitting room. Access to the gardens or patio. Whether visitors may take meals by arrangement or make tea.

PERSONAL POSSESSIONS: Can residents bring their own furniture? What security is required? What about insurance, televisions, radios etc. What can be done about labelling, storing and cleaning personal clothing? Can rooms be locked, and is there a lockable cupboard for the resident to keep their private things in?

TIMETABLES: Including details of regular social and recreational activities and outings, times of meals and arrangements to be made for outings, eg packed lunches. Details of local church services.

OTHER: For example who provides any necessary medical cover. Where to get information about fees and pensions and other money matters is also important. Not least, how to make a complaint.

Ways of telling

When it comes to the care of the elderly person, there are good and bad ways of communicating with relatives:

•"In the morning we get them up and wash them and toilet them. Then we feed them and toilet them again. They get three meals and a cup of tea between and we change them when they're wet. The TV is on for them to watch all the time, and we get them ready for bed after supper. The night staff are supposed to do them twice in the night to see if they are wet, or anything. Basically that's it." Day staff.

• "Hello... How is who?... Wait a minute... Oh, you mean the one who came yesterday in room one?... I've just done that room. She's a bit aggressive, isn't she? Don't worry, we'll take care of that." Night staff.

Why wouldn't you want to be a resident in that home? Frankly, I don't think you'd even want to work there. What is wrong?

When you visit the home that has been described in this way by one of the care assistants you may find, in the early morning, that some residents are still in bed, some are up and some are quietly getting themselves ready for the day. Of those who are helpless, some are being helped to get washed and to eat and drink, and some are resting quietly. The atmosphere is calm, but there is a lot of conversation, some laughter, and people listening to each other. People who need help to use the toilet are being helped discreetly. Now what is the difference?

It is the same place described differently. When relatives ask about the care provided, remember that the way you tell them can influence how much confidence they have in your capacity to care. We may be aware that some individuality is lost when people give up their homes, but you can show in your answer that you regard each person as special. When you ring up about your elderly relative late at night it would be better to hear:

• "Hello, Janice Jones speaking. Can I help you?... You want to know about your grandmother who has just come to us. Can you hold on a minute?... Yes, I can tell you I have just been in to help her settle for the night in her room. It takes a little time to get used to a new place, as I'm sure you know, but you can be certain that we will do everything we can to make her comfortable. Can I give her a message from you?...

Complaints

The same applies to complaints; there are good and bad ways of handling them.

When relatives complain they usually want at least one of three things:

• to get an explanation and an apology

• to get some recompense

• to draw attention to the fact that they are paying attention

Sometimes the first can be done quite easily:

"This is the third time I have visited and found that my mother does not have her dentures. What kind of place is this?"

It oils the wheels to start by saying that you are sorry that they have been upset in this way, and give an immediate explanation. For example:

– she keeps removing them because they hurt, and she is waiting for a dental appointment for some new ones
– she keeps leaving them in the toilet when she goes to rinse them after meals, and other residents pick them up (but you have had them marked and you are attempting to keep track of them).

You always have to tell the truth, but a good response includes the reason for the problem, and an indication of what is being done about it. This will often be enough to satisfy the person, but it is wise to let other staff know that the problem exists, especially the person in charge.

The question of recompense rests with the manager of the home, and the owners and insurers. Often people only go on to demand satisfaction if the first stage of

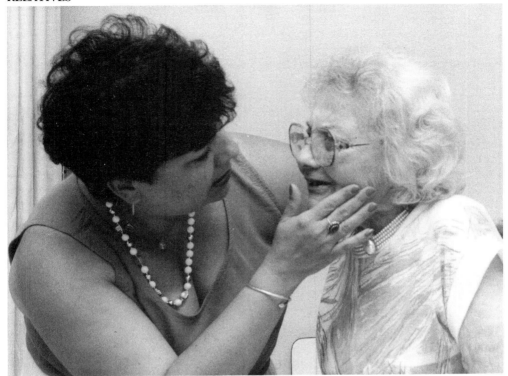

Welcome relatives' attention and try to involve them in caring and activities.

apology and explanation is handled badly.

The third item, drawing attention to the fact that they are paying attention, is one which staff often quote to each other.

"His niece was always in here going on about the food and his clothes and the way we cut his hair. Every little thing and she'd be running to the office. You can tell that she felt guilty about putting him here in the first place".

Some wise person has said that a lot of the anger expressed to staff by relatives is a result of the guilt feelings that they have. They get over their guilt by letting you know that you are being closely watched.

It is true that when you know that you have done something wrong you may take it out on someone else. It is a short step from slamming the door or shouting at the kids, to picking on a care assistant.

Unfortunately, some staff think guilt is the only explanation for dissatisfaction. Instead of examining what they do in the light of the complaint, they accuse the relative of feeling guilty, and dismiss the complaint without thinking.

Complaints are a good thing. They give you a chance to improve care. Maybe it takes someone's niece to have the courage to say that unless the cook takes a long holiday you'll all die of malnutrition. She might even know of a good barber who would come and do the hair. Her view may be valuable and her knowledge put to good use. Complaints also give you the chance to justify the care that you give:

• "I understand that you don't like me calling your mother by her first name, but I have asked her on more than one occasion, and that is what she tells me she prefers."

Give relatives confidence when you answer their questions. This means:

• listen very carefully to what they are saying

• give an answer if you can

• don't be afraid to say that you don't know

• make sure that they know that you will find someone who can give an answer

• make sure that the person in charge knows what kind of thing the relatives are concerned about.

Involvement

Some relatives want to get very involved in what is happening and some keep well out of the way. How do you feel about this? You might feel that the relative who stays away has dumped the resident, and doesn't care. But that may be wrong.

• "I don't go to see mum in the home. Well, the nurses all seem to know what they are doing and I only get in the way. I feel silly just sitting there – she doesn't know me any more. Do you think I'll end up like her?"

As a care assistant you know that old people who become demented appreciate company, even if they do not seem to know who it is. You can tell the relative this, and make sure that they do not feel in the way, as you rush about doing your jobs. Sons and daughters do worry about whether dementia runs in the family, and whether they will end up ill.

If you realise that they are possibly afraid, you can do the kind of thing that helps in an ordinary way. Let them get involved in the activities, make them feel wanted, listen to what they say and make sure that they can get to talk to the person in charge if they need to. Relatives can get involved in simple ways, providing a light entertainment, for example.

• "When our Sarah got married, dad brought the video and the slides to show gran at the home. Some of the other old ladies showed more interest than gran did, and he goes back once a month now to show his old holiday slides and pictures of us!"

Other relatives may seem to show too much interest. Always diving in and out of drawers, turning up at awkward moments and asking questions. But if someone has been taking care of her father at home for years, it can leave a great gap when he goes into a home. She is not feeling guilty, she is feeling lonely, and a bit at a loose end.

So welcome all the attention! If you are abrupt and avoid questions, they will multiply and come back in greater force. If you answer fully and pay a lot of attention to the person asking, you may find that they are satisfied and turn their attention elsewhere.

Suggest helpful things that the person might do. The really lonely person will love it. The interfering person may back off a little, or even better, find a good channel for their energies.

Support groups

When you are going though a difficult period, it often helps to meet with and speak to someone else with the same problem. There are practical as well as emotional problems associated with moving someone into care, and the help and advice that relatives can give each other is invaluable. They may meet by chance during visiting, but sometimes they form a support group. Often a member of staff will get it started in the first place, but then the relatives take it over and run it themselves. They may advertise on a notice board in the home, or by a letter to each new relative:

SEA VIEW REST HOME FRIENDS GROUP
MEETING 7PM LAST THURSDAY OF THE MONTH

Guest Speaker, Mr Bond from the College of Nursing on the subject of confusion and wandering
All relatives welcome

> *Dear Friend,*
>
> *We are a group of people who are united by having a relative living at Sea View Rest Home. We meet on the last Thursday of every month and have a short talk on subjects related to some of the problems of having a relative in a home. The tea and conversation afterwards usually lead to the next month's topic. We often ask a member of staff to attend. We have started a car sharing scheme for visiting and are planning a bus trip in the summer. We would be delighted if you would like to come and share both troubles and laughter.*
>
> *Betty Smith (Chair)*

Apart from the emotional support, the relatives group can do practical things to help each other and the residents. They are also a great help at the time of a death.

Death in the family

When one of your residents dies you will have a mixture of feelings to deal with. You may feel sorrow and loss, but also happy that you were able to make their last hours comfortable. You will also have to deal with the feelings of the family.

It is said that when an old person becomes confused and wandering, part of their personality dies. The daughter will say, "That's not my mother talking. She doesn't know me or her grandchildren. She would never say such terrible things."

Sometimes the old person will cease talking and responding long before they die, and just sit or lie in a dream-like state, unable to help themselves or talk. Relatives often say that it is as if they are already dead. The real person that they know and love has left, and the body left behind is just a shadow of the real person.

So when the old person eventually dies, it is a second death for the family. They may say that they feel it is better that the old person is dead, or that they feel relieved, because now they can mourn, although the old person died years ago when they became demented. Some people may be distressed because they were not visiting at the time of death. From a practical point of view it can be difficult if the resident is ill for a long time to arrange for the relatives to come at the right moment. The death may be sudden and unexpected, even if the person is old, so the relatives may have the shock of a telephone call or a message, apparently out of the blue.

If the relatives come to see the body before the funeral director takes over the arrangements, it helps them if you have shown respect by making the room and the body prepared. You may be asked to help the nurse wash the body and change the sheet, and you may comb and arrange their hair neatly for the last time.

With the room clean and tidy, some flowers and personal things still around, the relatives may wish to sit there alone, or with you for a few minutes, just thinking and talking about what has happened, and shedding some tears.

Helping with these last duties can be sad, but satisfying. You know you have done your best. Sometimes it is even worse if you come back after some days off and find that an old friend has gone, and there is someone else in the bed.

You can therefore understand how relatives feel. They used to visit you regularly and take part in the support group. They don't just lose an old relative, they may lose all the important friendships they had in the home.

This is why many homes make a point of welcoming relatives back after the funeral, for as many visits as they like. The experience of bereavement is something that they can share with the relatives group. The other residents also may appreciate the chance to talk to the relatives, to express their own condolences, and to continue friendships created through earlier visits.

Points to remember

As a care assistant you have a very important role to play in helping relatives to cope when someone comes to stay with you. The important things include:

1. Remember that everyone is different.

2. The way you describe things is very important.

3. Know what kind of questions will be asked.

4. Remember how to deal with complaints.

5. Welcome involvement, and try not to judge it.

CHAPTER 12

Managing ourselves

by Peter Watkins

Being open to your own feelings makes you a better carer • How to manage stress and build your own personal support system

We bring to our care of elderly people some knowledge of their disabilities and a range of general care skills, but, most important of all, we bring ourselves.

If much of what we feel, think, sense or experience is being kept hidden, we are unable to communicate much of ourselves to others. We are likely to find it difficult to engage with others in a warm, open, spontaneous way, and our care tends to be rather impersonal.

If, on the other hand, we are able to be more open to our feelings, thoughts, experiences and to share more of them with others, then this leads to the development of a rapport, enables trust to grow, and encourages other people to be open to us.

This is not to suggest that we need to be open books: I don't need to share everything, but enough of myself so that I can be experienced as a person in my caring role.

There will be times when what we feel and think seems incompatible with our caring role: when we feel irritated, exasperated, guilty, anxious, hurt, frustrated, sad or helpless. Everybody experiences these feelings; they are part of being human. What is important is that we learn to acknowledge them. Of course it is not always appropriate to express them as we experience them, and we may need to put them aside and deal with them later.

It is, however, important that we take the time to do this, because suppressed and repressed feelings do not go away but leak out in the form of bodily symptoms, irritable behaviour, poor concentration, impatience, or emotional outbursts.

Emotional repression tends not to be selective. We may for example have a tendency to repress our anger because we feel particularly uncomfortable with it, but repressing anger may mean that a lot of our more tender nurturing feelings become hidden and muted as well. Talking about our feelings to friends, people we work with, or at a staff support group allows us to discharge some tension.

A higher level of emotional release is achieved if we can not only talk about but openly *express* the feeling as well: to show our sadness, to ventilate our anger or to release our anxiety. To be able to discharge strong feelings is healing and restoring. It allows us to regain our emotional equilibrium.

Strong feelings

If we can achieve a greater degree of "emotional competence", then this is the most helpful skill we can bring to managing strong feelings in others. For example, if we can allow and accept our own anger and can appropriately control or discharge that anger, then we can accept and feel more comfortable with the angry feelings of a resident. We are then much more likely to be able to stay composed and manage such a situation calmly and effectively.

Personal Enquiry Exercise – This exercise will help you become more aware of how you manage your feelings.

Take a look at the following scenarios. Imagine yourself in these or similar situations. How might you feel?

• You are just about to go off duty when your senior asks you to help out with an extra shift tomorrow. It's difficult to say no. You agree reluctantly.

• A liked resident whom you have looked after for some time dies unexpectedly when you are on holiday. You hadn't got round to sending that card you promised.

• A resident behaves in a sexually explicit way when you are helping them to bed.

• A resident is loudly abusive to you and scratches you as you are helping her up.

• A resident wanders off from under your supervision and is returned some time later by a neighbour who complains about the old people not being properly looked after.

Now ask yourself: "What do I do with these feelings? Could I manage them differently or more effectively?"

Empathy

Being "emotionally competent" not only helps us to manage feelings in others effectively but also allows us to become more sensitively aware of the feelings and needs of others. Empathy is the human quality that enables us to understand something of another's experience and communicate that understanding in word and deed to them. Empathy is a skill that underpins a high standard of care. Cultivating this skill begins with inner empathy: understanding ourselves.

It can be difficult to empathise with people of a different generation, from a different background of experience from our own. But there is always more in common among people than there are differences. In empathising with elderly clients, we are drawing on human experience. We have all, for example, at some time in our lives , been lonely. We have all experienced loss and known dependence. Mining this seam of personal experience can allow us to respond helpfully and supportively to the experience of others.

Personal Enquiry Exercise – This exercise will help you explore your thoughts and feelings about dependence.

Sit comfortably, feet flat on the floor, read the instructions for this exercise, close your eyes and take a few deep breaths.

• Allow yourself to scan back in on a recent or significant time in your life when you have felt dependent. Recall the situation in detail: the setting, the events, who was there, what they said and did. How did you feel? Stay with the feelings or the memory of them.

• Now come back to the present time. It is sometimes helpful to stand up, stretch, maybe look out of the window and notice what is going on for a few moments to bring your attention fully out of the past.

• Now write a letter to a friend describing your feelings and experience of being dependent (not for posting!)

Often we don't know what we think and feel until we speak it or write it down. Be aware of any new understandings or insights that have come into focus about the experience of dependence during the exercise. How might you integrate them into your care of residents?

Self-worth

When we think about the helping/caring relationship, words like respect, valuing, accepting, trust, come to mind. For us to be able to express these qualities in our relationships, we must first of all be able to apply them to ourselves. The accumulated experience of being loved, appreciated, valued, respected as we grow up and grow older nurtures a positive self-image and allows our self-esteem to grow.

It is difficult to be nurturing to others and to feel confident in our work and in our lives if we do not have this basic sense of self-worth. A positive sense of self may not be constant: life crises major and minor can shake our self-image and self-worth and leave us feeling despondent and uncertain. But if our life experience has been predominantly one of loving care, acceptance and respect from others, then the wellspring of self-worth within us will remain uncontaminated, can be rediscovered and our confidence replenished.

Personal Enquiry Exercise – This exercise will help you become aware of the importance of supporting and valuing yourself.

• Reflect on some of the things you value, respect and appreciate about yourself. Make a list.

• Now ask yourself "Who in my life now appreciates me? What would they say about me?" Add these to your list. Be aware of any inclination to devalue these statements. Notice any negatives which surface among the positives and let them go. Celebrate yourself.

Acceptance

Accepting ourselves means that we also recognise our shadow. Alongside the strengths and qualities that we find pleasing and enjoyable are parts of ourselves that are less attractive. It is often these unaccepted parts of ourselves that we find unacceptable in others. If we find ourselves reacting strongly to, for example, selfish behaviour in others, it is well worth asking "What do I do with that behaviour in myself?"

It is often thought that to accept something means that it will stay the same. This is not so. Acceptance is the first step towards change. If I can acknowledge some less attractive part of myself and bring it out into the light of awareness, I can begin to see how it influences my behaviour.

Once something is known, the opportunity for change exists. If, for example, I remain unaware of my need to please and how that leads me to be patronising towards those in my care and to give help where it is not needed, then I cannot change.

Trust

Trust comes from knowing ourselves; being honest with ourselves; knowing what our strengths and weaknesses are. Trusting ourselves means that we can make choices, take decisions, initiate action for ourselves. We can rely on ourselves.

The foundations for a trusting orientation towards the world are of course laid by our very earliest relationships with our parents. If our needs are mostly recognised and met, if our discomforts and distresses are responded to, we absorb the message that people can be trusted. Later, if we are encouraged and helped towards self-reliance, then we absorb another important message: I can trust myself. This basic sense of trust runs through our lives and relationships. Without it we would be prey to many doubts, insecurities and uncertainties.

Many residents lose this trust in themselves as disabilities become more severe and the experience of failure increases. It is easy then to retreat into withdrawal and dependence. If we are to encourage and preserve the highest possible level of supported independence then we must trust our clients as they must trust us.

Taking care of ourselves

Taking care of others, particularly elderly people with psychological disabilities, can be demanding and stressful. The energy and resourcefulness that we have to bring to that helping relationship will depend greatly on our ability to take care of ourselves.

Professional helpers and carers are generally not good at this, not good at identifying and meeting their own needs. The challenge in our work can be stimulating. People often say they work better under pressure and it certainly seems to be the case that up to a certain point stress does improve performance.

Beyond that point, however, our performance begins to deteriorate. If we are subject to sustained stress at work or in our lives and do not adequately get rid of that stress, then we run the risk, not only of becoming inefficient and ineffective in our work, but of ill health (see graph). We can become so accustomed to living on the "down" slope that we become unaware that we are stressed until stress symptoms become so intrusive that we can no longer ignore them.

Personal Enquiry Exercise – This exercise will help you become aware of how stress affects you.

• Reflect back on a recent stressful period in your life. Focus on the way in which you were affected: physically, mentally, emotionally and in your behaviour.

Stress tends to have a diverse effect on human functioning. If you find it difficult to identify effects in particular categories, you may be ignoring important signs of stress in your life. Now compare your list with the examples in Table 1.

Stress, like beauty, is in the eye of the beholder. What we find difficult and stressful in our work, others may find less so. It is not so much situations that are stressful, but how we perceive them.

Take, for example, an elderly person in care who resists all approaches by staff. Try as they may, all they get is abuse. Some carers might find this behaviour very upsetting and stressful to deal with, perhaps seeing it as a rejection or as a reflection on their adequacy as a carer. Others may react differently, perhaps seeing the resistance and abuse in a less personalised way, interpreting it as the expression of the anger the client feels about his loss of independence.

Sometimes the stress we experience has more to do with some previous, perhaps distant, distressing experience that has been left undealt with, which mirrors in some way the current situation. In this case we might find that feelings of anxiety, anger, sadness can be re-stimulated by the current event. If we find ourselves upset unreasonably by a particular person or situation, it is useful to ask ourselves: "Who does he/she remind me of? When have I been in situations like this before?". The death of a resident may be particularly upsetting if it re-stimulates our own unfinished grieving for someone important to us who died, perhaps many years before. There is no time limit on undischarged grief; it may surface a very long time after the event.

Personal Enquiry Exercise – This exercise will help you identify key stressors, things you find stressful, in your work situation.

• Look at this list of stressors and decide which apply to you. Add other stressors not on the list that apply in your own work experience:

– having no say in what happens
– unexplained changes,
    poor communication
– death of a liked resident

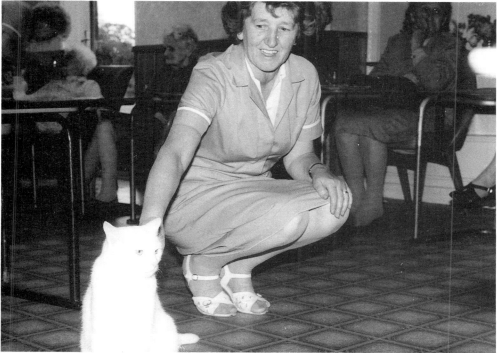

Carers are generally not good at identifying and meeting their own needs.

– having to deal with difficult behaviour (for example someone who is withdrawn, or aggressive behaviour, or wandering)
– lack of appreciation
– having to deal with unaesthetic and antisocial behaviour
– cynicism and negative attitudes in others
– routine work
– having to deal with complaining relatives
– breaking bad news
– witnessing the deterioration of residents
– heavy work load
– job responsibility unclear or unreasonable
– bad atmosphere amongst staff
– being criticised publicly
– having responsibility for very dependent people
– getting over-attached to residents **or** residents getting over-attached to me
– shift work

• Now rate the items on your list with high/average/low stress rating. Be aware of the number with high to average ratings that are present in your current work situation.

• Now ask yourself: What needs to change: The situation? The way I think about it? The way I react to it physically/emotionally? Perhaps all three?

• Now ask yourself: How am I going to do it? What resources do I have now that I could use? What new strategies could I adopt/learn that would be useful to me?

You may find it helpful to read to the end of the chapter and then return to this task.

Most of us have a range of strategies from the ordinary to the exotic that we use to manage the stress in our lives [Table II]. I use the term manage as opposed to cope with or resolve because the former implies treading water and the latter is often unrealistic: not all stress situations are resolvable. But what we can do is to manage the stressful situation and/or ourselves more effectively so that we stay mostly on the "up" slope, making stress work for us rather than against us.

Managing stress more effectively involves answering three questions:

What's the problem?
What do I want to do about it?
How am I going to do it?

We have so far been considering the first of these three questions. The second question involves considering what needs to change for me to feel under less stress and pressure.

We might decide that what needs to happen is that I need to be able to stay more relaxed in busy, pressured situations; or that I need to be able to leave work behind when I'm off duty; or that in amongst the demands of home and work I need some space and time for myself; or that I need to increase the support available to me; or that I need to reward and nurture myself a bit more, or that I need to say what I think and feel about the things that frustrate me.

We can think of these as desired outcomes which, if they were in place, would make a significant difference to our stress levels. Imagining how a situation might change realistically helps us begin to "climb out" from under the stress in our lives – to take charge of our lives.

The third question, "How am I going to do it?" translates these ideas into action. Let's take being able to stay more relaxed in busy pressured situations as our desired outcome. We might decide that one helpful piece of action would be to join a yoga class to cultivate a more centred approach to life, and we could also learn breathing techniques which could be used at times when we felt pressured.

We might also try building three short relaxation periods of five minutes each into our working day. Clearing your mind and letting the tension go from your body even for these for these short periods helps prevent over-stimulation. At home we could try an Alexander Technique "lie-down" during these five minute pauses. This is a valuable way of releasing tension and restoring energy. (It involves lying on the floor with two or three paperback books under your head and having your knees flexed and feet flat on the floor.)

Another strategy we may decide to adopt is to ask for more support from others or to speak to our senior about an unreasonable work load. For these last two strategies you may need to cultivate some assertiveness skills.

It is normally possible to generate a number of options to choose from. We might be able to make better use of ways of "de-stressing" that we have now but don't use often enough. We may need to learn or adopt new strategies.

Building up our repertoire of strategies for taking some of the stress out of life can lessen our dependence on unhelpful, potentially harmful ways such as excessive drinking, over-working, over-eating, excessively exercising, withdrawing, etc.

We need to keep in mind when considering how we might take better care of ourselves, how often intentions remain just that - intentions. It's helpful to ask ourselves: What is going to be my first move? When am I going to do it? Enlist the support of someone to help reinforce your commitment. Be aware of some of the things that might prevent you from getting started and keeping it going. Ask yourself: How could I reduce these obstacles? Remind yourself of the gains. Reward yourself for your successes. Learn from your setbacks.

Personal Enquiry Exercise – This exercise will help you become more aware of your support system.

Physical	Mental	Emotional	Behavioural
Headache	Forgetfulness	Discontent	Resisting change/ inflexible
Indigestion	Poor concentration	Anxious/worried	Cynicism
Tense, tight muscles, back /neck-ache	Difficulties with decision-making & thinking things through	Apprehensive a lot of the time	Absenteeism Talking a lot
Sleeplessness	Putting oneself down	Tearful	Overworking
Menstrual problems	Beating oneself up mentally	Hopelessness	Losing interest easily
Diarrhoea	Imagining the worst	Irritable, annoyed	Apathy, inertia
Tiredness, exhaustion	Changing one's mind	Angry more of the time	Withdrawn
	Confused, muddled		Destructiveness
Restlessness		Easily exasperated	
	Dreaming a lot		Drinking a lot
Cold hands & feet	Pre-occupied/ distracted	More despondent, sad, depressed than usual	Over-eating
Trembling			Insensitive, impatient with others
Jumpiness		Helplessness	
Frequency of passing urine			Avoiding people
Sweating		Resentful	Taking less care with appearance, diet, hygiene
Palpitations		High, excitable	Making mistakes
Tight breathing		Doubt/ uncertainty	
Pallor			Reduced commit-ment to work

EXAMPLES OF THE EFFECTS OF STRESS

Complaining a lot
Taking work home
"Busy" syndrome
"Indispensible" syndrome

Table I.

• Take a large sheet of paper. Represent yourself in the centre.

• Map out all the people and groups (also places, objects, activities, animals) that you experience as supportive. Put important sources of support close to you and less important ones further away. Draw in arrows to show whether support is one way or mutual.

• You may find in doing this exercise that you have a good, sustaining support system in your life right now. Conversely you may find it is somwhat limited. Ask yourself: Do I give out a lot but don't receive? Am I open to support? Is the support that I get helpful, ie not "rescuing", imposing or manipulative?

• Now ask yourself: What are some of the things I could do to strengthen my support system?

One of the universal strategies that enables us to feel more comfortable in the reality of our lives is the presence of support: the people, the places, the things in our lives that provide a support system from which we both receive and give help, comfort, encouragement, affirmation and advice.

The extent to which we develop and use a support system is partly determined by our attitude to support. For some people it may have negative associations with weakness, inadequacy, or with being smothered, while for others support is seen as an enabling, strengthening presence.

A supportive relationship is a great resource but it is unreasonable to expect one person to meet all our needs. The challenge is to develop and maintain a nymber of supportive relationships. We may, for example, unload a lot of our work frustrations on to a partner or a close friend, when what we need is the support of a trusted colleague who knows our work and can stand with us non-judgmentally in our frustrations and joys. Staff support groups can usefully meet this need.

Of course the best care teams are supportive to each other, but it can be helpful to set aside a specific time each week for the team to review their work, to share satisfactions and frustrations, to learn from each other's experience and to build good relationships between all members of staff.

Ways of managing stress more effectively

• Develop your problem-solving skills. People tend to deny, ignore or muddle through problems with a consequent increase in stress.

• Develop your assertiveness skills. A lot of stress arises from not being able to express your needs, put your point of view, make requests, say no.

• Be aware of how your thinking about stressful situations adds to your discomfort. Learn to use positive inner speech to challenge negative thoughts.

• Notice your breathing. Slower, abdominal breathing quietens and calms the mind and body.

• Learn the art of relaxation. Progressive muscle relaxation, the use of relaxing imagery, the Alexander Technique, etc.

• Nurture yourself: Get enough sleep, take care of your nutritional needs, etc.

• Have plenty of distractors in your life – conversation, pastimes, interests, exercise.

• Unburden to a friend or colleague. Talking about a stressful situation helps us to see it more clearly or differently. Having a good shout/cry/swear/laugh helps unload the distress and frees us for the next piece of living.

• Artistic expression (art, music, dancing) can facilitate release of tension.

• Develop and maintain a good support system: relationships that are a mutual source of help, advice, encouragement, affirmation.

Table II.

Points to remember

1. The most important asset we bring to the effective care of the elderly mentally infirm is ourselves. Knowing ourselves and taking

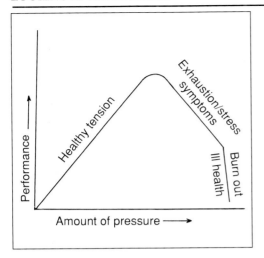

The effect of stress on performance.

care of ourselves pays dividends in sensitive, resourceful care.

2. Acknowledging our feelings and becoming emotionally competent helps us deal with strong feelings in others with more composure and resourcefulness.

3. Knowing ourselves a little better helps us become more empathic in our care of people, understand something of their experience and individuality, and reflect that understanding in our words and deeds.

4. Valuing, respecting, trusting ourselves enables us to feel confident in our role and to express these qualities in our care.

5. Listening to our bodies (the tensions and discomforts) and being aware of our psychological dis-ease: this helps us measure the stresses in our lives.

6. We can manage the stress in our lives more effectively by: changing the situation, changing the way we perceive the situation, changing the way we react in the situation.

7. Managing stress will help improve our effectiveness in work and life. It helps us stay off the down slope to burn-out and ill health.

8. Having a good support system is essential to our sense of well-being and enjoyment of life. We can also support ourselves through nurturing and valuing ourselves more.

Further reading

Bond M (1986). *Stress and Self-Awareness: A guide for Nurses*. Heinemann Nursing.

CHAPTER 13

Activities

by Theresa Briscoe

Do's and don'ts for success • Think small at the start
• Involve your local community • Ideas for every time of day • Special
events and outings • Activities with individuals

The care assistant and support worker are both in an ideal situation for planning and implementing individual and group activities.

It is YOU who are closest to the everyday needs of the resident.
It is YOU who will know the intimate details of the resident's behaviour over 24 hours.
It is YOU who will be able to incorporate individual projects and group activities in the home unit setting.

The first things that spring to mind when thinking of activities for the elderly are often bingo and World War II music, but activities do and can go beyond those! Activities can be as varied as art sessions to zoo visits. There are however some "do's and don'ts" for making a success of activities sessions.

DO

• Treat each resident as an individual. Even though their behaviour may at times seem very bizarre to you now, remember each has lived a full life until this time.

• Go at the resident's pace. If they get fed up after 10-20 minutes and you cannot finish the project, don't worry: there is always another day.

• Think small to begin with and there is less likelihood of frustration all round. Some people have always been loners, so to sit them down within a group could spell disaster.

• Plan ahead. Time set aside with friends and residents planning next week's programme is not only another activity, but also time well spent.

• Treat even the most confused as an adult. We are not to know the atmosphere they are picking up and it can be very distressing for relatives to see very childish activities taking place.

DON'T

• Don't forget to ask permission of your manager before you start. A little explanation of what you would like to do beforehand can often lead to a "yes".

• Don't forget the relatives and loved ones. Use them, their knowledge and love of your resident to help you plan and prepare. They are an invaluable source of help in your work.

• Don't put yourself or your resident ever at risk, be this at a cookery session or on an outing. Stay within the limits of your own expertise and knowledge.

Another don't: don't forget the community in which your place of work resides.

There are in most areas of the country branches of national organisations – Age Concern, Help the Aged, the Alzheimer's Disease Society, for example. Look in the telephone directory to find the nearest one to you, and ask what sort of help they give. Also be clear what you want from them. Do you want help to raise funds for equipment, or volunteers for special events?

Children's organisations are another great source of help. Often local Brownie and Cub packs are looking for ways to raise funds. Why not ask them to make your residents a project? It may also be possible to invite them into your setting – most elderly people like to see children and a great deal of sharing can take place.

If you have a large day area, why not invite local groups in to perform. Children's dancing schools and operatic societies are often great favourites. Some Women's Institutes or Towns Women's Guild groups have demonstrators on various topics, which may be suitable for the residents.

When involved in activities one becomes used to begging in the community. Not on street corners, but in local shops. Some chemists, newsagents and hairdressers will give testers, "end of ranges", away free.

Do take a formal letter with you from your manager to ensure respect in the stores, and always ask to see the manager or owner.

The activities

So – you asked permission, you have surveyed the area for free equipment, you have a few basic games and jigsaws, you know the residents well – now what happens?

Most workers in homes or units for the elderly tend to work shifts, therefore to help you choose the activities, suggestions have been placed in sectors: Morning, Afternoon, Evening, Night, Special Events.

Also, people tend to be certain types: up with the lark, only alive at midnight, etc. Although activities have been suggested in sectors here, they can of course be interchanged. For example, you could have a sing-along before lunch, or an entertainment in the afternoon.

Morning

Morning is a traditional "getting up" time. Make the everyday things of life as much an activity as a bingo session. Where appropriate suggest clothes to wear and where to sit afterwards. Don't assume everyone wishes to listen to daytime television. Try and arrange the day areas in group seatings, even though people may have a favourite chair. You never know, they might start to make friends in their group.

Often time for the care assistant is limited to actually getting on with the job in the morning, but certain activities can be planned and left for when there is an odd ten minutes.

Arrange for suitable newspapers and magazines to be around. When you are in need of a rest a "current affairs" session can take place, by sitting with a couple of residents reading the daily news, while you rest your feet. Some residents may be able to be left cutting out news stories from yesterday's paper for a weekly news board.

Leading on from newspapers, try and amass suitable books from the library and/ or memorabilia for reminiscence sessions. It is helpful if you know something of the period of your residents' youth, but not essential. Don't delve too deeply, keep the topics light hearted – fashion, transport, entertainment. The sessions again need not be formal, but 10 minutes sitting on the arm of a chair leafing through a book on old entertainers can be very rewarding for carer and resident.

If there are several lady residents why not make the hair care of the morning a special beauty session. If you consult with a friend you may be able to arrange to have a hairdressing session together. Treat it like a salon. Cups of tea, soft music and banter with residents. Simple plastic capes can be made and the session could include nail care and face massage.

This is also an ideal time for a volunteer to come in for an hour, say from 11am – 12am. Not only a new face, but it makes the session more of a treat. Don't forget the men – they will need a barber and nail care too.

Some residents may be able to undertake simple tasks, and often a small group can take place in the morning. Suitable activities include:

art – making backdrops for posters/calendars)

craft – making threaded chamois leathers/pompom balls

knitting – making squares/winding wool

sewing – making gifts like lavender bags/cushions.

Pop back every 10 to 15 minutes to ensure everything is going well, and the residents will feel less neglected.

The laying of the meal table is an activity in itself. Residents should be encouraged to volunteer on a rota of helping out with the general morning tasks. Some ladies will not have forgotten how to dust and clean. Men may remember how to clean shoes or brasses.

Afternoon

The afternoons for most care staff tend to be a little more relaxed, and therefore more supervised group activities can take place. It is also a time when volunteers are most likely to be able to come to help.

Be aware of residents' individual needs. Some may not wish to join in group activities and will need some supervision separately. Keep groups small, short in duration and simple. The following four need little equipment or preparation and can be achieved by mixed abilities.

Baking
An excuse to bake can be made at any time of the year: because it's the beginning of the month, because it's Saturday. Make ground rules to begin the session. For example: only staff to use the cooker, sharp implements not be left unattended. Simple recipes such as rock buns, biscuits, scones are easy to follow. Other items such as sweets and puddings can also be included.

Exercise
Simple exercise techniques can be learnt from a variety of sources. Ask the local hospital phsiotherapist to help start you off. Do ask your manager which residents will be able to take a full part in strenuous activities, as most elderly people have multiple medical problems. Simple exercises of raising and lowering legs and arms and moving from side to side in a chair – all to light music – can make the difference from someone being totally dependent to someone who can wash and dress themselves.

Gardening
This can take many forms and need not necessarily be out of doors. Arranging for fresh flowers to be delivered once a week and tending house plants can be as beneficial as tending borders.

But it is not impossible to garden outside, especially if there are a few tubs and beds on legs around. Try and choose plants which have a strong fragrance or different feel as the partially sighted and blind especially like this activity.

Sing-along

The weekly sing-along-a-Max (or Roy, or Des etc) can be boring for us, but often the elderly will remember tunes and music from yesteryear, better than modern times. There are now excellent cassette tapes and records available in High Street stores to help, but don't forget to ask the residents their choice. If some are in their middle sixties their heyday will have been the 1950s era of rock and roll, not Max Miller.

Evening

Evenings can be very busy times, especially if any of your residents are very frail and need attention at bedtimes. However, there are often one or two who like to stay up for as long as they can and may not just want to watch the television.

Although no one's wishes should be disregarded, it can be more beneficial if residents stay up for as long as they can, as they will often have a more peaceful night.

Again it is a time when some volunteers may be able to come in for an hour to help with individual residents, if time and staff are limited. A selection of games (old and new) is helpful for this time. Draughts, chess, even snakes and ladders have all proved popular. For the more agile of brain, cards and popular games based on television programmes are useful

For the more agile of limb, darts and indoor bowls are popular. There are special companies who deal with such equipment, but often a word with a local carpenter to make stands for playing cards or dominoes, the local publican for a darts board, can foster good relationships all around.

There are a number of excellent quiz programmes on the television at the moment, usually scheduled for times of the day when meals are being served or residents are not fully awake, or it's too noisy. A quick flick of switches on a video can mean half an hour of fun at quieter times, in the evening for example.

It may be possible to have some rivalry in the home, pitting women against men for example. Better still of course to devise simple quizzes oneself or with the aid of quiz books available at newsagents. The most popular are alphabet quizzes, proverbs and theme quizzes.

Quiet times in the evenings can also be used for reading to residents. This is especially useful for those whose sight is failing. Enquire at the local library or put out a plea to local churches to collect old books suitable for elderly people. Do not underestimate them however. Quite often a quiet "lavender and lace" lady will ask for a racy Mills and Boon love story! The most popular stories however tend to be the old classics – Jane Eyre, Pickwick Papers and poetry.

Music is another useful tool to have to hand at this time. Not the bawdy pub sing-along but more reflective music. The same sources for books could also be used for music, and possibly some Social Clubs, especially if it's records you require, as more clubs use tape cassettes. The choice again should be varied, from big bands to classical to jazz.

Again the video can be used to record musical programmes, but don't forget the radio. Many older people prefer this as sight and hearing deteriorates and they have often, in the past, only had a "wireless" to wile away the hours.

Night

There are often one or two people who cannot settle at night; perhaps they are up in the early hours of the morning, or wake extremely early. This is usually more a problem to other residents and staff than

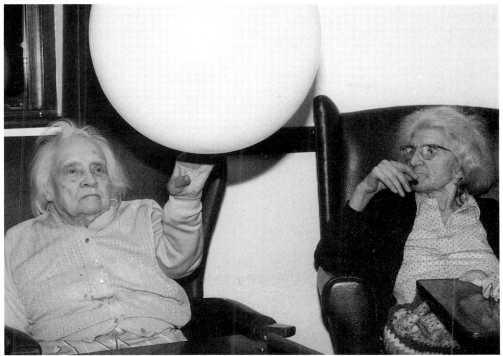

"Pass the balloon" is a simple but popular group activity.

to those concerned, although if one's sleep is disturbed it can mean a long night when worries come to the fore.

Night staff will sometimes say that the day staff always see the best of the residents and they do not get a chance to share in any activities, but this need not be the case.

Some of the quieter evening pursuits can be followed up at night. Like a child, many an older person can be lulled to sleep by someone reading a story or a passage from the Bible. A quiet game of cards or dominoes or a jigsaw can soon tire the restless eyes and mind.

For the more confused and those who tend to wander at night: always ensure they can be seen and the area is safe.

More mundane, but essential, tasks often fall to the night staff, but there is no reason a resident can not also join in. Do you have to fold plastic bags, fold napkins, slice carrots and beans? Why not let the resident help you?

Preparation work for daytime activities is also useful to have around. Here are a few examples:

1. Cutting pictures from old magazines.

2. Sorting out greeting cards.

3. Winding wool.

4. Knitting squares for blankets.

5. Sorting and cutting materials.

6. Shredding old stocking for fillings.

Some residents may be night people. They may have been so all their lives and at 70 plus would find it hard to change. Individual projects, for example completing a family tree, some basket work, some simple bed exercises or leafing through large print and picture books on a favourite topic will all make the night go quickly. The world does not necessarily have to shut up shop when the lights are dimmed.

Special events

Sometimes during the year opportunities arise to celebrate special events, or you can plan your own. This is another ideal time for introducing the community into the home, or taking the home out to the community. Below are listed six types of special occasions it is worth planning for each year:

Birthdays

Some elderly people do not want the passage of time to be marked, but for others, especially those who were unable to celebrate birthdays in the past because of financial constrictions, this can be a time for catching up. It can be as simple as a cake, a card and a bunch of flowers. Or it can be elaborate. How about a do it yourself kiss-o-gran (or grandad)? Encourage a local person or member of staff to dress formally and sing that person's favourite song at a party.

The party itself can mean cake for tea or a quiet candlelight supper for the birthday person and a friend or relative. If budgets do not run to too many parties, celebrate by "Star Sign" and you have an instant theme.

Outings

In the warmer months it is nice to get out. Do not let the lack of suitable transport deter you, although if you have a minibus it's a great help. Check the legal requirement and procedure before commencing planning in your home/unit, as some may require a trained nurse to accompany residents.

Younger volunteers make good wheelchair pushers. A minibus means the world is your oyster. Zoo visits, carnivals, Christmas lights are all popular. Often though an elderly person wants to just reflect. So a quiet stroll to watch the seasons change, window shop or watch the children play, can have as much meaning as the most elaborate outing.

Entertainment

As mentioned earlier, outside entertainment is often a welcome intrusion into the residents lives. Make the choice as varied as your local community allows. The most popular entertainers are singers, piano/organ players, anything to do with children, magicians. Comedians do not often go down very well, neither do playlets as they demand too much concentration for most residents, but for those who can appreciate such events, their moment could come when planning outings.

Festivals

Every calendar month has a festival of some nature to celebrate. Some are religious like Easter; some full of memories, like Remembrance Day. Some are full of pageantry, like the Queen's birthday parade; some are fun, like August bank holiday.

It also helps when planning activities to have a theme for the month. Here are some suggestions. January – New Year. February – Valentines. March – Spring. April – Easter. Collages can be made, visits planned, or television programmes watched, parties held, groups formed.

Fundraising

Some residents, especially those in private homes, will see no point in fundraising for themselves. However, fundraising can be encouraged to help other causes and can also make life worthwhile for the residents. For example: making blankets for Oxfam, a white elephant stall at the local church fete. We all like to feel wanted. If the residents can see they are still of worth, they are still wanted, they will hopefully live life to the full to the end.

Individual projects

Some elderly people are loners. It may be because they always have been, or circumstances over the years have made it so.

Finding out as much as possible of a person's background history is not prying, it's caring, to enable you to give good individual attention. Try and think of one thing which is special to each person you care for at work. It may be they worked on a farm, as a policeman, or have never been abroad. Suitable individual projects, with the help of family and friends if possible, can then be pursued.

Worthwhile

The aim of individual and group activities is not just to occupy the residents' time or to make our job easier. The main aim should always be to make that person's life worthwhile to the end.

As suggested earlier, we all need to feel wanted, to have a purpose in life, to feel it's all worthwhile. This is no different whether we are eight or eighty. Yes, activities will make our working lives more enjoyable; they will mainly however, maximise the life that is left for our residents.

Points to remember

1. Plan ahead. Be ready for next week's event this week.

2. Think small. Working successfully with one person is far better than being frustrated in a group of six.

3. Think of individuals. It is so easy to generalise about residents, but each has her/his own personality.

4. Think adult, not child. Although children's games are useful, adapt them to adult thinking.

5. Use the day. Events can be spread through out the whole day, don't try and rush everything in the morning.

6. Make life normal. Think of the everyday events some elderly people attend and adapt them to your residents' needs.

7. Think of special times. Use the festivities, celebrations and events of the year to plan special projects.

8. Use the community. Don't take all the strain: there are a lot of untapped sources of help in the community.

9. Use voluntary agencies. Survey the area and see what services are available and make them aware of you.

10. Smile. Even when the going is tough and boring and repetitive, a smile to them can help you as well.

CHAPTER 14

Psychiatric emergencies

by Ian Hicken

• What might happen • Prevention is the best strategy • Your own feelings and behaviour • Policy and procedures • Know each individual • Practical steps in an emergency • The Mental Health Act

An emergency is an unexpected occurrence which requires immediate action. This chapter will attempt to describe the principles of the care and management of the elderly mentally infirm person when an emergency arises. It will provide you with immediate practical guidance on what to do if you are faced with an emergency situation and outline some of the legal aspects which could be involved.

For most of the individuals in your ward or unit it will be the first time in their lives that they have experienced mental health problems. By far the majority will be suffering from a recent deterioration in their ability to function intellectually, however it is possible that some of your patients/residents have a previous psychiatric history.

Depression, anxiety, thought disorder and alcohol abuse are just a few examples from a range of health problems which your patient/resident may have previously experienced. The type of emergency situation which you may be faced with will be equally diverse. To prepare you for every eventuality is impossible, but there are several principles which are common to all emergency situations.

What might happen, and why?

The psychiatric emergency is a relatively rare occurrence; effective teamwork can often prevent a situation arising. Disturbance of mood can be a result of "external" and/or "internal" triggers, it is only when these triggers go unnoticed that it could result in a possible emergency.

Examples of external triggers could include an inappropriate approach by staff or visitors, one which makes the patient feel insecure or threatened. A recent admission could trigger off feelings of anxiety and insecurity which in turn could exacerbate confusion, disorientation and mood disturbance. Unfamiliar surroundings, change of routine, loss of independence and security could cause the patient/resident to react in an untypical manner. The loss of a loved one or friend could have an impact on the individual's mood; they may experience shock or depression.

Examples of internal triggers could include an abnormal reaction to medication, withdrawal from alcohol or tranquillisers (common following admission). Acute toxic confusional states may be caused by constipation, build-up of drugs or malfunction of internal organs.

Previous personality has an obvious role to play in determining what reaction might result. In most instances a combination of external and internal triggers will affect how the person reacts. It can be a very useful exercise to begin to identify behaviour as part of a sequence of events rather than something that happens spontaneously. More often than not a psychiatric emergency is the consequence of this sequence of events:

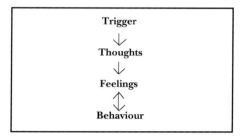

An example of this sequence of events might run as follows:

Mrs Jones is admitted (trigger) into care because of her inability to manage at home due to her confusion and disorientation. She does not understand what is happening to her (thoughts) which in turn makes her feel anxious, insecure and frightened (feelings). As a consequence when confronted by a nurse who tells her that "this is now your home" (trigger) she becomes increasingly anxious and frightened. This results in her attempting to leave the unit to go back to her home.

When once again confronted with the fact that this is now her home she becomes acutely agitated and disturbed. She lashes out at the member of staff (behaviour) and does not respond to gentle coaxing or distraction.

Depending on the severity of her behaviour, this could be classed as a psychiatric emergency. It would be extremely useful if as a carer you could predict this possible sequence of events and therefore go part of the way to prevent it happening.

Examples of emergency situations which could occur are as follows:

1. Violence and aggression.
2. Deliberate self harm or attempted suicide.
3. Extreme, acute agitation, anxiety or fear.
4. Acute thought disorder, delusions (false beliefs).

When considering psychiatric emergencies it is important not to exclude physical emergencies. These are covered fully in Chapter 15, but there are certain situations which may be made more likely due to mental health problems. These could include:

1. Increased risk of falls and accidents.
2. Hypothermia (lowering of body temperature).
3. Choking on food and drinks.

Let us briefly look at these examples in more detail.

1. Increased risk of falls and accidents

An elderly person who has mental health problems could be more at risk than usual due to a number of reasons. Their mental health problems may necessitate medication which may subdue or tranquillise, and this in turn would have an effect on their mobility and reaction time.

An example of this could be the elderly man who is on sleeping tablets because he frequently wanders at night. The tablets could impair his ability to climb stairs or negotiate a change in the level of a floor – a step or the beginning of a carpet. He may trip up and because the tablets have sedated him, his reaction time may also be impaired. The result would be that he is unable to prevent a fall.

2. Hypothermia (lowering of body temperature)

Decreased intellectual capacity could impair the individual's ability to judge a situation: an example of this is not being able to distinguish between hot and cold. An electric fire or a hot drink may not be recognised as being dangerous.

Hypothermia is when the body's temperature falls to a level which is dangerous and could lead to death. An elderly person with mental health problems might not be able to judge whether or not an extra layer of clothing was needed, in or out of doors.

3. Choking on food and drinks

Choking can be a very real problem for elderly people for several reasons. Badly fitting dentures or an inability to chew food properly could cause a resident to get a lump of food stuck in their windpipe. Deterioration in the body's ability to function properly may cause swallowing problems, and this can be made worse when a person is on medication that causes sedation.

What can I do?

For a nurse or carer, the prospect of having to face an emergency situation can be a frightening experience. With appropriate guidance and support you will feel more confident and able to cope such an emergency arise. First and foremost it is important to be honest with yourself about your own thoughts and feelings. Remember the sequence of events which was described earlier; this can apply equally to the way you react to a situation. For example:

The trigger: Patient/resident admitted with a previous history of violent behaviour.

Your thoughts: I am scared of this person.

Your feelings: (a) Physical: butterflies in stomach, tension, dry mouth. (b) Psychological: anxiety, fear, apprehension.

Your behaviour: Avoid this person as much as possible.

This pattern of behaviour is very common and a natural reaction when faced with uncertainty. Every nurse or carer, irrespective of grade or position, has felt this way at some time during their career. To acknowledge these feelings is the first step in overcoming your fear. Once you can recognise what effect your thoughts have on your feelings and behaviour you will be able to acknowledge to yourself that this is real for you. To keep these thoughts and feelings to yourself can be a destructive process which will cause you to feel stressed and unhappy in your work. Just as important, your patient/resident will not be receiving the care he/she requires.

Talking about your thoughts and feelings to more experienced staff is essential; this should be an ongoing process in any care setting. Throughout your working day you will be faced with unfamiliar scenarios which may need discussion to help you clarify your thoughts. Do not feel that it is a sign of weakness to admit these feelings, it shows maturity and strength of character if you can talk about them openly and honestly.

In many care settings it has become routine to have staff meetings where opinions, anxieties and thoughts can be explored and discussed, but to admit to these feelings in front of the rest of the staff can be an intimidating prospect. If you feel that you cannot voice your fear in this setting perhaps another solution would be to talk to a senior member of staff at an appropriate time.

Communication between staff members is essential when considering the management of an emergency situation. Knowing who you work with and how they work will strengthen your team and in turn will inform you of what is expected of you as an individual. It could be that a member of your team has found a way of defusing a particular situation or that he/she may have developed a rapport with a particular patient/resident which would enable you to gain insight into the reasons for that person's behaviour.

FIRST STEPS
1.Acknowledge thoughts and feelings.
2.Identify sequence of events and your

resulting behaviour.

3. Voice your anxieties and concerns.

4.Communicate with team members.

Policy and procedures

Most hospitals and homes have a book which outlines policies and procedures relating to specific incidents. As a carer you should have access to these documents and become familiar with their content.

A policy is a statement of intent which details a plan or course of action for specific situations, and a procedure is an action or set of actions necessary for doing something. Policies and procedures in care settings should cover emergency situations, eg, violent patients, accidents, fire, compulsory admission of patients and grievance procedure. Ask a senior member of staff to guide you through these policies and procedures and to explain anything you find difficult to understand.

Individuals

Once you have recognised your own needs you can then begin to develop your skills in recognising your patients/residents needs.

Knowing who you are caring for is crucial to the wellbeing of the individual. It may be stating the obvious to say that your patient/resident is a unique individual with a unique personal history, an individual with their own set of beliefs, morals, customs and terms of reference, but without keeping this in mind at all times there is a possibility that your approach will become generalised and inappropriate.

Knowledge about the individual's life style, beliefs, customs, family and social network will inform you about a person's character and about their possible concerns and anxieties. Information about the circumstances which led to the admission is also very important.

Sources of information:

1. The patient/resident
2. Relative/friends
3. Case notes
4. Other staff members

Talking to the individual is important: getting to know them well will enable you to plan your care and approach. Relatives and friends are a rich source of information: what seems "abnormal" or "strange" behaviour to you may be usual for the individual.

Case notes will detail family, social, medical and psychiatric history and will outline the circumstances leading to admission. However, as with any other information about patients/residents, it is confidential and there could be information contained in the notes to which you will not have access. Check with a senior member of staff first before reading any information.

Previous psychiatric history can be an indicator in determining risk. Someone who has a history of attempted suicide is more likely to try again, as opposed to someone who has never attempted to harm himself.

Other staff members are also a valuable source of information. They may have previous experience of caring for the person or they may have noticed a particular behaviour pattern of which you need to be aware. It is common for people to confide in other support staff such as a domestic, kitchen help, chiropodist etc, so including these members of staff in case discussions can be appropriate.

Observation of the patient/resident is important in determining mood and behaviour disturbance. Are they more withdrawn? Has their ability to communicate altered? Their appetite increased or decreased? Is their sleep pattern disturbed? All these are important indicators of mood disturbance.

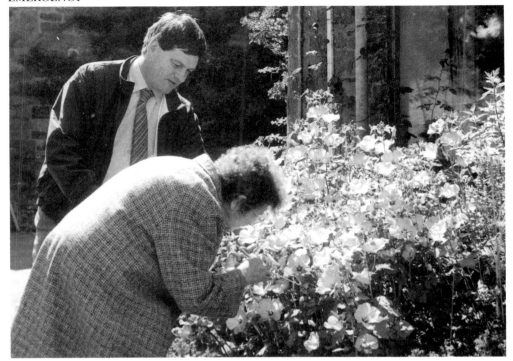

Getting to know an individual well will help you spot important changes in mood or behaviour.

Any information you obtain or observations you make should be passed on to a senior member of staff in order that care planning and delivery can be monitored and evaluated.

If something happens

There are several practical steps you can take to minimise any difficulty you may face if an emergency occurs. Because you are part of a team you have a responsibility to ensure that your colleagues are aware of your whereabouts at all times and that you are aware of theirs. It would prove somewhat tedious to constantly inform your colleagues of your every movement, but if you are about to carry out your duties in an isolated part of the unit or if you intend to leave the unit for any reason, your colleagues should be informed.

Alarms

Being familiar with alarm systems, how they work and where they are, will ensure help is close at hand.

Procedures for managing emergency situations should contain important telephone numbers of whom to contact and when. These telephone numbers could indicate how to contact:

1. The Police
2. Ambulance
3. Fire Brigade
4. Emergency doctor/medical help

Having a working knowledge of the telephone system will prevent you becoming flustered if you need to summon help through a complicated phone network.

The environment

A safe environment is especially important when caring for elderly mentally infirm people. Not only will it reduce the risk of accidents to residents but it will also minimise potential dangers to staff.

If you are caring for someone who has psychiatric problems, an appropriate location in which to care should be considered. The resident may need closer observation and supervision, therefore a room which is near to the focus of staff activity is more suitable than a room at the other end of the unit.

The room should be comfortable but uncluttered; having unnecessary objects around which could be used as weapons or missiles is unwise. Placing somebody who is potentially disturbed near windows, sun lounges or balconies could prove dangerous. Many patients/residents will have visitors who bring gifts, toiletries and other creature comforts such as alcohol or cigarettes and matches. Advice about such gifts should be considered: alcoholic drinks, matches, tablets and sharp objects such as razors and nail files can all complicate the safe care and management of the disturbed resident.

How do I respond?

Your immediate response if something did happen would depend on the type of emergency which occurs, but there is a golden rule to remember:

• Remove danger from the resident if at all possible.

• If this is not practical, removing the resident from the danger should be considered.

For example, Mr Smith is sitting quietly at the dining table when suddenly he becomes disturbed and starts shouting and throwing things. He is hearing voices (auditory hallucinations) telling him that he has been locked up and people are trying to kill him. He believes that the staff are all against him and out to get him (delusion).

Your response could be as follows:

1. Stay calm: panic will not help.

2. Summon help: use an alarm, shout for help, ask other patients or visitors to seek a member of staff.

3. Ensure your own safety and the safety of other residents.

4. Remove potential danger such as hot drinks, teapot, excess furniture (this should be done with discretion – you do not want to add to someone's paranoid beliefs).

5. Attempt to defuse the situation by talking to the patient, but if it is obvious that he will not respond to this do not attempt to stop him until help arrives (don't risk injury trying to prevent crockery or furniture being broken).

6. Be prepared to offer help to experienced colleagues. This will depend on the situation. You could be called upon to help restrain Mr Smith if necessary, make a telephone call or fetch assistance.

An important point to stress is that your colleagues will have had experience in managing these emergency situations and will guide you through. Afterwards you may need to talk through the events; this will help you understand what has happened and why, and will assist you in future if a similar situation occurs. It can be upsetting to witness such situations and therefore consideration should be given to your emotional needs and those of the other patients or residents. Talking about your feelings always helps.

Legal aspects

Mental health problems can be very disabling for older people. They may result in increased risk of neglect, self injury or abuse. The individual concerned is at risk of becoming a danger to him/herself and others, but there are laws in force which aim to protect the rights of the mentally ill individual.

In days past a disturbed patient could be detained in a secure environment against their will for an indefinite period of time. Inhumane conditions prevailed and the individual concerned was at further risk of neglect, injury and abuse.

Today, however it is a different picture. As long ago as 1890, regulations concerning the rights of individuals were conceived and enforced. The Mental Health Act 1959 revised in 1983 (England and Wales) is the legislation governing the rights and regulations for people who experience psychiatric problems. Similar acts apply in Scotland and Northern Ireland but they do vary slightly from English and Welsh counterparts.

Protective framework

The Mental Health Act is designed to serve the best interests of the individual and society as well as giving the caring professions a framework in which to work, protecting their professional competence and discretion. Anyone who is admitted into hospital is in legal terms an informal patient: that is to say they are there by choice and in theory could take their discharge whenever they so wished.

There are circumstances when admission to hospital for assessment and/or treatment would be appropriate and there are times when patients/residents already admitted on an informal basis need to be detained against their will. This is where aspects of the Mental Health Act can be enforced.

Application for compulsory admission is made by a social worker who has specialised training, or a close relative (this is defined in the Act). Admission is then recommended by one or two doctors depending on which type of admission is required. The same applications can be made while a person is in hospital or care but the procedures can differ. Under clearly defined circumstances a registered nurse can "detain" a person against their will for up to six hours, but the nurse must then follow very comprehensive guidelines and ensure appropriate authorities are informed. What follows is an overview of the most commonly used sections of the Act:

Section 2: Assessment order

Reason – Compulsory detention in hospital for assessment followed by treatment, for reasons of their own safety or for the protection of others.
Who applies – Nearest relative or approved social worker and two doctors (one GP and one psychiatrist).
How long – 28 days.

Section 3: Treatment order

Reason – Mental illness, mental impairment or psychopathic disorder which warrants detention in hospital for the interest of health or safety of patient or others.
Who applies – Nearest relative or approved social worker and two doctors, one GP and one psychiatrist.
How long – Six months initially.

Section 4: Emergency order for assessment

Reason – Urgent need to be admitted because of mental disorder.
Who applies – Social worker or relative plus one doctor.
How long – 72 hours from time of admission.

Section 5: Detention of informal patient already in hospital

Reason – Urgent need to detain patient because of danger to self or others.
Who applies – Nominated doctor.
How long – 72 hours.

Section 136: Place of safety order.

Reason – Individual in a public place who appears to be suffering from a mental disorder and to be in immediate need of care and attention.
Who applies – Police constable.
How long – 72 hours.

The Mental Health Act is complicated but very necessary to protect the rights of individuals. You will not need to know the complexities of it but to have an awareness of the basic principles will help you understand why it is used and how it can benefit the individual in care. When someone is compulsorily detained in hospital there are very strict procedures to follow; regular and accurate records must be maintained at all times and the patient must be informed of their rights.

The Mental Health Act makes provision for the individual to appeal against any such application for compulsory admission or detention. Information on this process should be available for the patient/resident and their next of kin. Further clarification of the Mental Health Act may at times be necessary for you to fully understand it. This is perhaps best sought as you experience it: being able to relate its application to an individual you know will help put it into perspective. Talking to a senior member of staff will help you understand the reasons why it is used.

Summary

When considering the management of a psychiatric emergency, it is not possible to describe what to do in every situation. The circumstances surrounding each emergency will be unique and diverse; each one will demand a different course of action and intervention. This chapter has attempted to explore various basic principles surrounding the management of a psychiatric emergency. Most emergencies in psychiatry can be avoided and easily controlled; being part of a team is essential in order to achieve this. Learning from each other, sharing feelings and ideas is very important. As you progress in your career you will become better skilled and your confidence will increase. The psychiatric emergency will become an event you manage effectively and efficiently, in a way that best promotes the self respect and well being of the elderly mentally infirm people in your care.

Points to remember

1. The psychiatric emergency is a rare occurrence.
2. Communication: teamwork aids prevention and effective management.
3. An emergency is a sequence of events; it does not happen in total isolation.
4. Get to know the people you care for as individuals.
5. Become familiar with policies and procedures.
6. Maintain a safe environment at all times.
7. Know how to summon help.
8. Ensure your own safety and the safety of your other patients.
9. If possible remove danger from the patient.
10. Stay calm. Afterwards talk to a senior member of staff about your experience.

Resources
Mental Health Act Manual, edited by R. Jones. Sweet and Maxwell (1985).

CHAPTER 15

Accident and emergency

by Teresa Mearing-Smith

• The aims of First Aid • What to do in an emergency or following an accident • Common conditions and useful action the care assistant can take • When to call for help

Sooner or later, as you work with elderly people, you will find yourself having to cope with an emergency. There may be an accident; someone may suddenly become very ill and distressed; or they may collapse and become unconscious. Whatever the situation, there are important and simple principles of First Aid which you can apply, while waiting for qualified help to arrive.

First Aid

The aims of First Aid are:

- To preserve life
- To prevent the condition worsening
- To help recovery

No one will expect you to make a precise diagnosis, but you are in the ideal situation of knowing the residents, what medical conditions they may have, what drugs they are taking, and whether or not, for instance, they have a tendency to fall, or suffer from fits, chest pain or breathlessness.

The following steps will help you to act in the right order of priorities:

Assess the situation

You must appear calm and confident. This is important not only to help you to cope, but also to prevent fear and anxiety spreading to other residents or staff who may witness the emergency. If appropriate you should take charge, and make use of any other residents who are well enough to fetch another member of staff. You must ensure the safety not only of the casualty, but also of yourself and other residents. There is for instance no point in a second resident slipping on the wet patch on the floor on their way to get help.

Decide what has happened

There are no marks for getting the answer right, but it will be helpful for both yourself and others who may take over to know exactly what has happened. Ask other residents or relatives what they saw or heard, or even smelt. Of course, if the resident can tell you herself, that makes life much easier.

Now have a look at the resident. What

can you see that might give you a clue. Has the resident fallen and hit her head, or cut herself? Is she conscious? What is her colour like? Then use your hands gently to remove any harmful object, undo clothes to get a better look, or feel her skin or limbs. Is she hot? Cold? Sweaty? Or is one limb swollen, indicating a fracture?

Obviously you must get the right balance between finding out what is wrong, and preventing further deterioration or doing unnecessary harm. If you remain calm and confident it is unlikely that you will do the wrong thing.

Treatment

The first and most important steps are to ensure the person has:

- An open airway
- Adequate breathing
- Sufficient circulation

The **Recovery Position** is important here. This is similar to the position in which you would put a very frail or dying person; on her side with the upper leg bent and resting forwards to take the weight of the lower half of the body while the upper half rests forwards on the upper arm (see figure 1). The importance of this position for someone who is unconscious is that the head is on its side and there is less obstruction to breathing. The tongue is less likely to fall backwards, and vomit or mucus is less likely to collect at the back of the throat. You may need to place a resident in this position; certainly if their breathing becomes noisy this is the best position for them to be in.

The next important step is to **dress any wounds** using a simple gauze dressing and micropore tape, or gauze held on with a bandage. If bleeding has not stopped you will need to apply pressure on the wound until it does. More serious large wounds or fractures can be covered with a clean (non-

fluffy) cloth, but dressing should be left to a trained nurse.

Put the casualty in the correct position. I have mentioned the recovery position, but a conscious patient may well wish to sit up, propped slightly forwards. She will probably tell you which position is most comfortable. If the situation appears serious and you have taken the preliminary steps I have listed already, it is probably better not to move the person more than is necessary.

Perhaps most helpful of all in this situation is the care assistant who **remains calm and has a calming influence** on the victim and others around. **Be sympathetic**, reduce pain and discomfort as far as you can, handle the person gently to prevent more harm or pain, and protect them from cold and damp.

It is your responsibility as the first person on the scene to **make sure the resident is not left in an unsafe condition**. Therefore you should call the doctor, or officer in charge or other staff as appropriate and inform the relatives if necessary. This is where your account is important, for other people whether trained or not will want to know what has happened, and what treatment, if any, you have given. If you have managed the situation yourself, you should enter the details in the Kardex or Day/Night Book as appropriate.

When to call for help

It is a good idea to discuss with the officer in charge and other staff, what the home's policy is on calling for help in an emergency. You should know whether you are expected to call the doctor or an ambulance yourself, or whether other trained staff or the officer in charge will do this. You should know which residents often have little "turns" from which they recover quite quickly with basic help, and which residents have more serious conditions. If you are unsure of what to do, it is far better to call for help than to struggle on by yourself.

Do you know?

Telephone:
Where all the telephone extensions are
GP's number(s)
Nearest Accident Centre number
Officer in charge or other staff at their home (if appropriate)
Where to find residents' relatives' numbers

How to switch off:
Gas
Electricity
Water

Fire:
What the Fire Drill is
Where the Fire Extinguishers/Fire Blankets are

Medical:
Where the First Aid box is
What drugs each resident is taking
How to open the drugs cupboard

It is worth finding out all this *before* the emergency happens!

Now I will describe some emergency conditions and how to cope with them.

Breathing

Choking: Try to feel in the mouth for the obstruction (eg food or false teeth) and remove it. To do this, gently open the mouth and use two fingers to sweep around inside, but be careful not to push the object further in. If a resident turns blue while eating, puts a hand to their throat and cannot speak, use the Heimlich manouvre (Figure 2).

Asthma: You will know which residents suffer from this condition and how badly it affects them. A sudden deterioration may be helped by an inhaler if the resident has one; occasionally they may need oxygen. Try propping them up in a chair or in bed, talk calmly, offer a drink to sip and call for further help if there is no improvement.

Winding: This occurs with a heavy blow or fall onto the upper abdomen. Sit the resident down, loosen tight clothing and gently massage the stomach. This treatment normally works well.

Hiccups: These can be very distressing if prolonged. Holding the breath, taking long drinks or breathing in and out of a paper (not plastic) bag often stops the attack, but seek further advice if the hiccups persist for more than three hours and the resident is distressed.

Circulation

Shock: This can happen if blood or other fluids are lost from the body, (from severe cuts, burns or diarrhoea and vomiting). The resident will be weak and faint, pale, cold, and sweaty, and may be breathing faster.

If you think shock is the problem, you must seek further help, but you can reassure the resident, lie her down on her back with her head on one side and elevate the legs, cover with a blanket and loosen clothing; but do not give anything to eat or drink until advised to.

Fainting: This is a brief loss of consciousness caused by insufficient blood reaching the brain. It may occur as a result of sudden pain, a fright or sometimes hunger. Lie the resident down. Tell her to take deep breaths and loosen any tight clothing. Make sure there is plenty of fresh air; sometimes a sip of cold water will help.

Angina and heart attacks: Angina is a temporary problem, usually brought on by exercise or stress; it causes pain in the chest and sometimes the left arm. There may

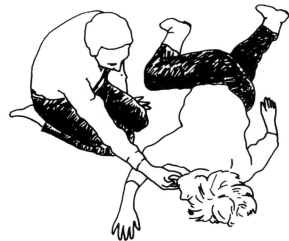

The Recovery Position: when you have positioned the casualty's body, readjust her head to make sure her airway is kept open.

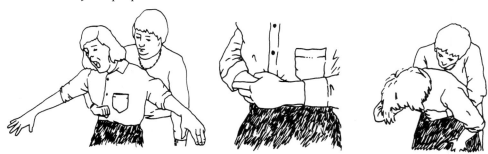

The Heimlich Manoeuvre. 1. Stand behind the choking victim and clench one fist, thumb towards her stomach. 2. Hold this fist tight with your other hand – it should be placed under the ribs, between the navel and breastbone. 3. Pull sharply inwards and upwards, three or four times (pushing the upper abdomen against the lungs to force air violently upwards).

also be sweating and difficulty in breathing.

Get the resident to rest by sitting or lying propped up, and loosen clothing. Here your knowledge of the residents is important: if you know that she suffers from angina and has little tablets or a spray to put under the tongue (Glycerin Trinitrate) or other treatment for an attack, give it or find someone who can.

A heart attack is a blockage in one of the blood vessels carrying blood to the heart muscle and may look like severe angina (therefore use the same treatment) or it may cause death, either sudden or preceded by severe chest pain.

Summon help and make sure that other residents are not distressed by what is going on. Put the person in the Recovery Position, whether or not there are signs of life. Sometimes, although apparently dead, a person may start breathing again and this position will aid their recovery.

Bleeding: One day you may discover one of the residents in a pool of blood. This may have resulted from an injury, perhaps to the scalp or shin.

Don't panic! A little blood goes a long way and the resident may have spread it around herself, either in confusion or in an attempt to clear it up. Aim to control the bleeding and prevent the wound from becoming infected. So first quickly wash your hands and find the First Aid box or supply of cotton wool and gauze. If small, clean the wound itself either by gently placing under running water or with cotton wool swabs, then cover the wound up with a piece of gauze and clean the surrounding skin. In this way you can tell exactly how big the wound is and what other damage if any has been done.

If you think you are competent to put on a suitable dressing then do so. If you are unsure then ask a trained nurse to put on the bandage. If the cut is more serious then call for help straight away. If the bleeding persists, press firmly on the wound for five to ten minutes, or until the bleeding stops, and elevate that part of the body if you can.

Nose bleeds: These may cause the loss of a lot of blood which can be swallowed or inhaled, and could cause vomiting and/or difficulty in breathing, so the resident may be very frightened at the sight of all the blood she has lost.

Remain calm and sit her down with her head forward over a bowl or basin. Pinch the soft part of her nose just below the bone and get her to breath through her mouth avoiding swallowing, coughing, spitting or sniffing; carry on pressing for ten minutes then release. If the bleeding persists carry on for another ten minutes. If after thirty minutes the bleeding still has not stopped, then summon help. If the bleed has been a severe one it is probably a good idea for the resident to sit propped up in bed for a few hours, and avoid any exertion.

Varicose veins: These may bleed quite dramatically, and frighten the resident, so remain calm, apply pressure on the site of bleeding, and elevate the leg. Lay the resident on her back, remove any clothing over the leg and press directly on the vein with either your fingers or the palm of your hand over a dressing. Make sure there are no tight stockings or suspenders constricting the leg higher up. If the bleeding is not controlled quickly then get help.

Bruising: This is caused by bleeding just under the skin which causes a bluish purple mark, and sometimes swelling. The elderly bruise very easily so you should know how to help. If the injury has just happened, raise the injured part, if possible, and place in a comfortable position, apply a cold compress (ice-pack – or a bag of frozen peas is ideal). Once the acute stage is over, it is important that the resident is encouraged to move, so as not to become stiff.

Nervous system

Concussion: This is caused by a fall or a blow to the head. Injuries of this sort often cause unconsciousness, if only for a few minutes. If the resident comes to very quickly, place her in a chair or lying down and comfort her. She may well feel sick or actually vomit, so be prepared.

If she is unconscious place her in the Recovery Position if possible, and seek help. Head injuries in elderly people do not always follow the usual pattern, so always tell a trained member of staff if you think the resident has suffered such an injury.

Stroke: This is caused by the blood supply to part of the brain becoming suddenly cut off, either because of a clot or a haemorrhage into the brain. This is another condition that is common in elderly people, and is often associated with high blood pressure.

In its mildest form, a stroke causes weakness on one side of the body or face or difficulty in talking, which may last for half an hour or less, and is followed by complete recovery. More serious is the weakness that is very severe and shows only minimal improvement after days or weeks.

The most serious form of stroke is associated with loss of consciousness and total inability to move one or the other side of the body: death commonly follows.

Your role here is to help and comfort the resident who is probably very frightened and confused. You may not be able to understand her, but she may well understand you. Get her to a safe comfortable position if possible.

If she is unconscious, place her in the Recovery Position or at least in a position where she is not a danger to herself or others. Those who have had a stroke usually cannot move themselves and are a dead weight, therefore if you want to preserve your back, do not attempt to move them alone: get help!

Epilepsy: The disease results from abnormal electrical discharges in the brain and causes involuntary movement of the body, usually lasting no more than five minutes, and followed by confusion or a dazed feeling. You should know, if any residents in the home suffer from epilepsy, what may cause the attacks, and how they are best treated. While the attack continues you should help the resident into a safe position on the floor (unless they are in bed at the time). Loosen any tight clothing, do not try to restrain and do not put anything in the mouth.

Allow the spasms to stop, and the resident to regain consciousness, and then help them into bed or a chair until fully recovered. There is no need to call for an ambulance or the doctor immediately unless the fit lasts for more than fifteen minutes, several fits occur in short succession, or the resident has not had a fit before. The fact that a fit has occurred should be noted in the records and the doctor informed in due course.

Diabetes: This is caused by the body's inability to use sugar properly, and is common in the elderly. Most diabetics will have treatment either with diet or tablets rather than insulin injection. It is unlikely that a diabetic with dietary control alone will suddenly deteriorate, but conditions such as chest infection or stomach upset could upset the blood sugar levels. Those on tablets, however, may become suddenly ill if they have not eaten (and therefore become very *low* in sugar) or if an infection or other illness causes the blood sugar level to become *high*.

Low sugar (hypoglycaemia) causes paleness, sweating, rapid breathing, trembling and confusion. The treatment is to give the person a sugary drink or boiled sweet. Symptoms should improve dramatically; if not, seek help quickly. High blood sugar (hyperglycaemia) should be suspected in any diabetic who has become unwell. Drinking excessively and passing water very frequently are the first signs, followed by deep breathing and drowsiness. This is serious and needs immediate attention.

Injuries to bones, muscles and joints

As you will know from experience, elderly people are often unsteady on their feet, perhaps from arthritis, a previous stroke, painful feet or poor vision, and are therefore liable to fall and injure themselves. Older ladies in particular often have brittle bones (osteoporosis) and can break a bone very easily.

If you suspect that one of the residents has fallen, it is important that you report this to the officer in charge, as the resident herself may not remember what has happened. Sometimes an elderly person becomes confused or takes to her bed, with no complaints of pain or a fall, but a broken bone, especially in the hip, must be suspected.

A fractured hip bone (head of the femur) is a serious injury. It typically causes the leg to appear shorter and to be turned outwards, sometimes with swelling and pain around the hip, but this may be difficult to see. In fact you may be amazed to find that an elderly person has walked on a broken hip with very little complaint. Normally a doctor would need to confirm the diagnosis, but the home may have a policy of calling the ambulance immediately if the diagnosis is obvious. An operation is normally needed, and it is remarkable how quickly elderly people can recover from this, and are back on their feet within a few days.

Another common fracture is of the wrist (Colles fracture) caused by falling on to an outstretched arm. This is normally easy to see, as there is pain and swelling at the wrist, and sometimes an obvious "bend" in the bones. Again this requires hospital treatment; usually the results are very good, but there may be permanent stiffness, swelling and pain.

Other bones may break, such as the collar bone (which normally heals by itself with the arm in a sling) and the ribs which can be very painful, but again heal by themselves. The shoulder can dislocate in a fall and require hospital treatment. Although elderly people often fall and cut their heads, fractured skulls are uncommon.

Sprains and strains: A strain occurs when a muscle is overstretched and torn by a sudden movement, while a sprain occurs at a joint when it is suddenly wrenched. There is swelling, pain and stiffness. Treatment for these injuries is rest, ice (a bag of frozen peas is particularly good), compression with a thick layer of cotton wool and bandage followed by elevation.

These may not all be possible; for instance you may find it difficult to elevate a leg when there is bad arthritis of the hip. It is also important that an elderly person does not get put into bed for days on end, as they then risk developing pneumonia, pressure sores, constipation or incontinence, and will have difficulty in getting mobile once again.

Cramp: This occurs when a muscle suddenly goes into spasm, and can be very painful. It often happens to elderly people during sleep. Gentle stretching of the muscle and massage will help. You need to straighten out the leg or the toes carefully and gently massage the area that hurts.

Burns: It is often difficult to assess the seriousness of a burn: if in doubt, call for help. Any significant burn requires medical attention, and any burn affecting the leg, arm, chest, back or head requires hospital treatment. Elderly people are less able to stand the shock of a burn, and will need hospital treatment more often than fitter, younger people.

You can help further damage occurring in a minor burn by cooling, either by placing the area **gently** under running water or soaking the skin in cold water. Hot, wet clothing should be removed as quickly as possible as in a scald (which happens with wet heat such as steam, hot water or fat). Cooled dry burnt clothing should be left in place.

Once the burn has been cooled it may only need a simple dressing to protect it. If a blister forms, do not burst it, as infection is then possible, delaying healing. New skin will grow under the blister, and over the next week or so the skin of the blister will gradually dry and peel off. If a blister is large and does break, then you will probably need to ask a trained nurse to dress it.

Hypothermia: This develops when the body temperature falls below about 35 degrees Centigrade (95 degrees Fahrenheit). One would hope that elderly people living in residential care would not suffer from this condition, but a resident could well fall out of bed and be unable to attract attention for some hours. In this case it will be obvious that she is cold, and the possibility of hypothermia, like that of a stroke or a heart attack, must always be considered.

Re-warming should be done gradually, with any wet clothing removed first and the resident placed in bed in a warm room. You must ask for further help.

CHAPTER 16

Rules and regulations

by Deirdre Wynne-Harley

*• The law that affects you • Registration and inspection of homes
• Keeping accurate records • Residents' rights • Complaints • Health and
safety at work • Employment legislation*

This chapter is about the law and mentally frail people in residential care and nursing homes.

The most important thing to remember is that whatever dependency, disability or illness your residents suffer from, they are individual people first and foremost with all the normal rights of citizenship. Carers have a duty to protect these rights and ensure that residents' autonomy and civil liberty is not infringed by the care and treatment given.

The legislation which regulates life and work in homes falls into three broad categories:
– registration
– residents' rights
– employment and health and safety

Each of these topics is discussed below.

NOTE: The legislation quoted applies specifically to England and Wales. Requirements in Scotland and Northern Ireland are similar and the acts are listed at the end of the chapter.

The legislation – what it says

The Registered Homes Act 1984 governs residential care and nursing homes. This Act, together with the regulations and guidance, sets out the requirements for registration and operation of homes. Some homes are "dually registered": that means they have both beds for residential care and for people who need nursing care.

The law requires that all care homes with more than three residents and all nursing homes regardless of numbers must be inspected and registered by the appropriate authority. Until 1991 this has normally been the local social services department for residential care and the health authority for nursing homes. Under the 1990 Community Care Act new multi-disciplinary inspection units will take on this responsibility for residential homes. They will still be locally based and work closely with the health authority.

The registration covers client groups and the numbers of residents who may be cared for in the establishment. Sometimes registration will be refused or cancelled; in these cases the proprietor may appeal to the Registered Homes Tribunal, which will either confirm the decision of the registration authority, uphold the appeal against this decision, or vary the conditions of the registration. The registration authority must comply with any directions made by the Tribunal.

How it works

1. Starting up

Anyone wishing to open or take over an existing home MUST apply for registration.

2. The Certificate

When a registration certificate is granted, the home must abide by its conditions as to number and type of resident/patient. When registration authorities consider applications, they will specify certain criteria regarding the suitability of the applicants and the premises. They will also issue guidelines about the services and facilities to be provided and the level of staffing. Criteria and guidelines will be based on the 1984 Registered Homes Act and Regulations, *Home life: a code of practice for residential care,* the NAHA *Handbook on Registration and Inspection of Homes (1985)* and guidance from the Department of Health. The certificate must be displayed in a prominent place.

3. Inspection

Inspection is an essential element of the registration process and includes continuing checks on standards. The Registration or Inspection Officer will visit the home at least twice a year and one of the visits is likely to be unannounced. These visits ideally provide opportunities for residents and staff to meet and talk to the officer from the inspection unit. The manager of the home will receive a written report after the inspection. The registering authority will also require that the home continues to comply with the demands of the fire department, environmental health department and the building regulations. These requirements will be reviewed from time to time and the registration officer will check that they are up to date.

4. Records

When the home is registered and operating normally, certain records must be kept, and be available at all times for inspection by authorised officers of the registration authority.

These records must include:-

• A statement of the aims and objectives of the home, of the care and attention to be provided in the home and of any arrangements for the supervision of residents, which has been supplied to the registration authority and has been agreed with that authority. In practice this means that staffing levels, therapeutic and rehabilitation facilities and services agreed must be provided.

• A daily register of all residents (excluding persons registered or persons employed at the home and their relatives) which must include the following particulars:

(a) the name, address, date of birth and marital status and whether the person is the subject of any court order or other process

(b) the name, address and telephone number of the resident's next of kin or of any person authorised to act on his behalf

(c) the name, address and telephone number of the resident's registered medical practitioner and of any officer of a local social services authority whose duty it is to supervise the welfare of that person

(d) the date on which the resident entered the home

(e) the date on which the resident left the home

(f) if the resident was transferred to a hospital or any other home, the date of and the reasons for the transfer, and the name of the hospital or home to which the resident was transferred

(g) if the resident died in the home, the date, time and cause of death

(h) if the resident is an adult who is subject to the guardianship of a local social services authority, the name, address and telephone number of that authority and of any officer of the authority whose duty it is to supervise the welfare of that resident

(i) the name and address of any authority, or organisation or other body which arranged the resident's admission to the home

- A case record in respect of each resident shall include details of any special needs of that resident, any medical treatment required by the resident, including details of any medicines administered and any other information in relation to the resident as may be appropriate, including details of any periodic review of the resident's welfare, health, progress

- A record of all medicines kept in the home for a resident and of their disposal when no longer required

- A record book in which shall be recorded the dates of any visits by persons authorised to inspect the home, that is any registration or inspection officer, fire officer or environmental health officer

- Records of the food provided for residents in sufficient detail to enable any person inspecting the record to judge whether the diet is satisfactory, and of any diets prepared for particular residents

- A record of every fire practice drill or fire alarm test conducted in the home and of any action taken to remedy defects in fire alarm equipment

- A statement of the procedure to be followed in the event of fire

- A statement of the procedure to be followed in the event of accidents or in the event of a resident going missing

- A record of each person employed at the home to provide personal care for residents, which shall include that person's full name, date of birth, qualifications, experience and details of that person's position and dates of employment at the home, and the number of hours for which that person is employed each week

- A record of any relatives of the registered persons or of persons employed at the home who are residents

- A statement of the facilities provided in the home for residents and of the arrangements made for visits by their parents, guardians, friends and other visitors

- A record of the fees applicable from time to time including any extras for additional services not covered by that scale and of the amounts paid by or in respect of each resident

- A record of all money or other valuables deposited by a resident for safe keeping or received on the resident's behalf, specifying the date on which such money or valuables were deposited or received and the date on which any sum or other valuables was returned to a resident or used, at the request of the resident, on the resident''s behalf and the purpose for which it was used.

This may all seem to be very complicated, but is usually made easier by the use of standard recording systems.

Care staff will often be involved in providing some of the necessary information. Through recording in a day book their observations of the residents' health, activities, appetite and so on, a valuable contribution may be made. It is very important to ensure that any accidents to residents or staff or incidents such as a missing resident, or sounding of the fire alarm (whether this is a false alarm or not) are recorded. It should be standard practice in all homes for staff to exchange information when shifts change, so that staff coming on duty understand any notes in the incident book or in the residents' records.

Residents' rights

It is important to remember that the legal rights of residents in residential care and nursing homes are exactly the same as those of any other citizen, and staff must always bear this in mind in their day-to-day duties. It is all too easy when caring for people to diminish an individual's basic rights without being fully aware of doing so. This happens most commonly through the use of forms of restraint, through medication and health care, by withholding information, and most of all by the erosion of choice in daily life and activities.

Sometimes it will be necessary for decisions to be made on behalf of an individual who has become incapable of doing so themselves. The legal position is often unclear as physical and mental conditions may change dramatically or almost imperceptibly over a long period. There are often also variations, ups and downs which can create uncertainty about a resident's true mental state.

The common law test of "capacity" is to the effect that the person concerned must at the relevant time understand in broad terms what he is doing and the likely effects of his action. Thus, in principle, legal capacity depends upon understanding rather than wisdom: the quality of the decision is irrelevant as long as the person understands what he is deciding.

The Mental Health Act 1983 itself contains three different approaches. The first in Parts II and III governs compulsory admission to hospital and guardianship, the second in Part IV governs consent to particular forms of treatment for mental disorder, and the third in Part VII governs the management of property and affairs.

Whatever the situation, care staff should never make decisions or even assumptions about a resident or patient's mental capacity without guidance from the home's medical advisers.

Managing finances

Many older people have informal arrangements for the management of their finances and property. Often these will be handled by a close relative or friend. Sometimes a solicitor or bank manager will act on their behalf.

On no account should care or nursing staff become involved in residents' affairs.

Where an individual has no one to assist with their affairs, the registration authority should be asked to recommend someone to act as his or her agent. There is an increasing number of advocacy groups which offer specially trained volunteers to help elderly people in this way. Social services, Age Concern and Citizens Advice Bureaux will usually know of local advocacy schemes.

Some residents will be under the jurisdiction of the Court of Protection and all their affairs, property and money will be managed through the Court of Protection. Increasingly, as people get older, they are making Enduring Powers of Attorney (EPA). This means that they give someone else the power to represent and act for them in matters of property and finance at some time in the future if the need arises. Then if they become unable to make decisions for themselves the EPA is registered with the Court and the named representatives takes over. No one connected with the home should be appointed an attorney.

Restraint

Physical restraint should never be used in residential care in any form – including restraining chairs. If it appears that restraint is necessary, the home is clearly not an appropriate place for that resident to be, either in terms of staffing or in the facilities and environment provided. Restraint in this situation is an assault on the person and consequently could give rise to legal action against the manager or member of staff involved.

In nursing homes restraining chairs should only be used in exceptional situations. They should never be a substitute for adequate staff cover. The use of cotsides is more likely to cause accidents than provide protection as residents may fall while trying to get out.

Consent to treatment

Admission to a home does not change an

individual's right to choose his or her own general practitioner. Neither does it change the rules on consent to treatment. The law provides that no medical treatment can be given to any person without his valid consent. Any breach of this rule will result in the person concerned being liable to legal proceedings. For consent to be valid, the patient must be given information about the proposed treatment or medication, be competent to give consent and give consent voluntarily. If the resident has difficulty in understanding or communicating in English, every effort must be made to find an interpreter to explain the purpose and effect of the treatment. When a resident or patient is not able to understand because of their mental state, treatments prescribed by the GP or consultant must be in the best interests of the individual but keeping in mind any strongly held views they have expressed in the past.

Medication

No drugs except simple "household remedies" should be given without a doctor's prescription. Whether residents retain and administer their own medicines or these are kept by the manager, proper arrangements must be made for safe keeping. All medicines must be in individual containers, clearly labelled with the name and dosage. When held by the home, they must be administered ONLY by a responsible person authorised by the manager. Staff responsibility does not include insisting, forcing or tricking residents into taking medication. If residents refuse, this should be noted and the GP informed. Medication must not be used for control or punishment. As with restraint, inappropriate or forceful administration of any medicines is in effect a physical assault.

Access to information

Changes in the law over the past few years have given people greatly increased rights to know what is said about them in personal records. This applies to residents also. Therefore, subject to adequate safeguards and counselling where necessary, individuals should be able to see the records about themselves kept by the home. Any decision to withhold information should only be taken at a senior level in the organisation and the reason for doing so explained to the satisfaction of the registration authority. All residents' records should be kept securely with strictly limited access.

Residents' finances are often a matter of concern and a recent amendment to the legislation [Residential Homes (Amendment) Regulations 1988] requires that homes keep detailed records for each resident of any money or valuables (including social security benefits) received on his or her behalf and indicating how this was spent or disposed of. Residents or their representatives must have access to these records.

Complaints

Residents and their families have a right to know how and where to contact the registration authority if they wish to make a complaint or discuss some matter which has not been resolved between them and the management. Information about who to contact must be displayed clearly, preferably near to the registration certificate.

Health and safety and employment legislation

The Health and Safety at Work (etc) Act 1974 obliges all employers to ensure as far as reasonably practicable the health and safety at work of all employees.

Accident prevention

Safety is also covered in the 1984 Registered Homes Regulations. This states that "the person registered shall, having regard to the size of the home and the number, age, sex and condition of the residents, take adequate precaution against the risk of accident, including the training of staff in first aid". Inspectors from registering authorities will enquire into accident prevention arrangements, when making visits. The home will also receive occasional visits from the health and safety or environmental health officers who are responsible for enforcing the Health and Safety at Work legislation. Properly authorised inspecting officers have legal rights of access to homes.

In matters of safety, staff must be alert, observant and careful. Accident prevention in residential homes, as in our own homes, is often a matter of common sense. Legislation and special precautions will be ineffective if equipment is not used correctly or defects reported. All accidents in the house or grounds, however minor, affecting residents, staff or visitors should be recorded in detail without delay. Any witnesses should also make and sign written statements. This is very important and should be done immediately.

Policy statement

Where five or more people are employed, the employer must have a written policy statement regarding safety at work, including arrangements for carrying out that policy. All staff must be made aware of this policy and any subsequent changes.

For staff in residential and nursing homes, special risks may be associated with lifting and helping residents to move. These risks are to residents as well as staff and illustrate the importance of having a clear safety policy and appropriate accompanying arrangements for training. Every home must have at least one first aid box clearly marked. All staff should know where this is kept.

Emergency procedures

Emergency procedures must also be clearly stated and understood by all staff. These should cover

– procedure in the event of a fire
– procedure in the event of accidents
– procedure if a resident is missing

Food hygiene

Food hygiene is another aspect of safety which may involve care staff, especially in small homes where job specifications are more flexible.

The Food and Drugs Act 1985 and the Food Hygiene (General) Regulations 1970 apply in residential and nursing homes and it is the responsibility of the manager to see these are observed. Staff must be aware of regulations which affect them directly, like the requirement for wearing clean washable over-clothing when handling, preparing and serving food. Any members of staff who have kitchen or dining room duties should follow the basic rules of hygiene displayed in the kitchen. The Food Safety Act 1990 now requires that *all staff* who handle food attend approved training courses in basic hygiene.

Health

There are also health requirements and staff must inform their employer if they are suffering from or are a carrier of:

– typhoid
– paratyphoid
– other salmonella infections
– amoebic dysentry
– bacillary dysentry
– any infections likely to cause food poisoning, eg septic cuts, boils, burns, sore throats or nasal infections.

Any of these infections will have to be reported to the local medical officer for environmental health who will advise the person in charge about necessary precautions.

Your employment

Employment law is very complex. Both employer and employee have rights and duties and these should be clear to both parties when the appointment is made. The Employment Protection (Consolidation) Act 1978 provides that all new employees (who work over 16 hours a week) should be given a written statement of terms and conditions of employment within 13 weeks of starting. This statement must give the names of employer and employee and the date when the employment starts. It must also detail:-

– job title
– rate of pay and whether this is weekly or monthly
– hours of work
– holiday entitlement, including public holidays
– arrangements for such pay
– notice period
– pension schemes

Information about disciplinary rules, grievance procedures, and persons to whom application should be made if the employee is dissatisfied with any disciplinary action against him should be available in the contract or a separate specific reference document.

If any terms or conditions change, the employee must be informed in writing within one month of what such changes are.

Trade unions

In law every employee has a right to membership of an independent trade union; they also have an equal right not to belong to a union. This is regardless of whether or not the employer recognises the union. An employer may not prevent or deter employees from being members of independent trade unions or compel them to join one.

The employer is free, however, to choose whether or not to recognise a union. "Recognition" means the employer recognises the right of the union to represent its members in collective bargaining. The relevant legislation is The Employment Act 1980.

Rehabilitation of offenders

Under the Rehabilitation of Offenders Act 1974 a person who received a non-custodial sentence of not more than 30 months, and is not convicted during a specified period, becomes a rehabilitated person. His conviction then becomes "spent", in other words it is regarded in law for most purposes as never having occurred.

There are, however, certain types of employment (listed in the 1975 Order) where this does not apply, provided that when asked about previous convictions, the person is told that by virtue of the Order spent convictions must be declared. The exceptions include occupations concerned with carrying on an establishment required to be registered under the Registered Homes Act 1984.

Data protection

Many homes now use computers for keeping personal records of staff and residents. Under the Data Protection Act anyone storing personal information about other people must register with the Data Protection Registrar. The onus is on the computer users to declare themselves. As with the residents, staff have a right of access to information about themselves held by the employer.

Conclusion

This chaper has highlighted the areas of legislation which are most likely to affect care staff directly or are concerned with the registration of the home.

There may be occasions when a member of staff becomes aware of acts or incidents which breach some aspect of the law. These may be minor and perhaps arise from a genuine oversight or of a much more serious nature. Whatever position an individual holds, they have a duty to residents and colleagues to take some action. The first course would normally be to discuss the matter with the head of home and in the case of a safety hazard to alert colleagues until the danger is removed.

If the matter appears to concern the work of a senior colleague and affects the residents' well being, the advice of the registration officer should be sought. The registration authority has a duty to investigate any possible offences against the Registered Homes Act. Similarly serious concern about matters of health and safety should be reported to the Environmental Health Officer if no remedying action is taken by the Head of Home.

Fortunately staff are rarely in a situation where they have to report incidents or practices in a home. However, if this does happen, they should not be deterred from taking the correct course of action through fear of the consequences.

Work with people who are mentally frail or have dementing illness can be very stressful and it is often easier to provide a regime which assumes a generally low level of ability in all residents. But each resident is a different person and, however ill, will respond differently. By treating each one individually, however severe their dementia, their rights as citizens will be protected and maintained to the greatest degree possible. This will also be seen to enhance the work of the carers and the quality of life of the home as a whole.

Main legislation quoted

Registered Homes Act 1984 and Regulations 1984, amendments 1988 (England and Wales).
Nursing Homes Registration (Scotland) Regulations 1988 (came into force November 23 1988 and covers both residential and nursing homes).
Health and Personal Social Services order (Northern Ireland).
Health and Safety at Work (etc) Act 1974 (whole of UK).
Employment Acts 1980, 1982, 1988.
Employment Protection (Consolidation) Act 1978 (whole of UK).
Food Safety Act 1990 (whole of UK).
Guidance:
Home life: a code of practice for residential care, published by the Centre for Policy on Ageing, 25-31 Ironmonger Row, London EC1V 3QP. Tel: 071 253 1787.
NAHA Handbook - Registration and Inspection of Nursing Homes, 1985, published by the National Association of Health Authorities.

Points to remember

1. Residential care and nursing homes must be registered and work within the terms of their registration.
2. Proper resident records must be kept on the premises and any accident or incident should be recorded immediately by care staff in the day book.
3. Residents' property must be safeguarded and a record kept of all valuables deposited for safe keeping.
4. Staff of homes should never take responsibility for residents' finances or accept a power of attorney.
5. Physical restraint of residents is an assault and may give rise to legal action.
6. Residents and their families must be given information about how to make a complaint.
7. Think safety – staff should always be alert and observant.
8. Be aware of all the emergency procedures.
9. Staff have a duty to report accidents or incidents which they believe are wrong or illegal.
10. However frail the resident, their civil rights must be protected. Personal and nursing care should not reduce their rights or dignity.

CHAPTER 17

Opportunities for training

by Richard Banks

How to select the right form of education and training for you • How to use the National Vocational Qualification System to ensure that your skills, knowledge and understanding are recognised for employment and career progression

This chapter is intended for all people involved in personal care, including those who care for the client group which is the subject of this book, elderly mentally infirm people. Education and training are matters for constant attention as we gain a better understanding of how best to work with other people, and the changing ways care is provided. What sort of training and education are suitable for you will depend on your individual needs. The way in which education and training are provided also has to be organised to match the time you have available and the type of education or training that suits you. It is also important that the skills, knowledge and understanding you gain, by whatever means, should be properly recognised and recorded. This is important whether you intend to improve your work practice, have your present skills identified or carry on to further qualifications.

You're in charge

Therefore there are two main aims to this chapter. To show you:

1. How to select the right form of education and training for yourself.
2. How to use the National Vocational Qualification (NVQ) /Scottish Vocational Qualification (SVQ) system to ensure that your skills, knowledge and understanding are recognised for employment and career progression.

In thinking about how to find and select the correct education and training in personal care, the things people consider generally fall into the following categories:

How can I get help in working out what I want?

How can I identify the skills, knowledge and understanding that I have now - so I know my starting point? (As a general rule people find that they can do, and know, more than they imagined).

What is the end result that I want from this education, training and assessment?

What are the practical issues to be solved, such as finding time?

How can I be sure the education and training will be organised in ways that help me to learn and not repeat negative experiences of the past?

Will I experience discrimination? Or will anti-racism and anti-discrimination be part of the content and part of the experience?

All of these are legitimate concerns, but until recently people have often felt unable to ask about them because of the difficulty in gaining any education or training opportunities at all, or the fixed nature of some courses. A way of looking at this problem is to separate three issues about education and training that are often confused:

1. The opportunity to obtain education and training.

2. The assessment of individuals.

3. The requirements of employers.

Confidence

The NVQ/SVQ system has separated assessment from education and training. This means people requiring education and training can approach the matter with a greater sense of confidence and assertiveness. It is now the education and training providers' task to ensure that what they offer is what is wanted in terms of success in assessment, the needs of the workplace and the needs of individuals.

There will still be potential for conflict between individuals and employers, possibly about what a person needs to be able to do in order to do a particular job. The standards upon which the National Vocational Qualification system is based, and the awards given, are approved by employment interests (the Care Sector Consortium) but are not attached to any particular job. So they do provide a basis but cannot in themselves solve any conflict between what an employer will spend on education and training and what the staff as individuals or as a group want. The care sector trades unions (who are represented on the Care Sector Consortium) have information about NVQs/SVQs and will be able to offer some assistance to members.

The outcome of your learning must be clear. With the introduction of NVQ/SVQs for care staff there is now a developing system which enables those employed or contemplating employment in personal care to gain recognition for their skills, knowledge and understanding, even if they have received little or no formal training. This is a major change: there have been some excellent courses, but no proper national recognition of the work involved in social care.

The actual existence of these awards is however only part of the change; the way people are assessed for these qualifications is another. NVQ/SVQs are not courses; people will be able to gain an NVQ/SVQ without taking any formal training. This is possible because the qualifications are based on the idea of COMPETENCE IN THE WORK PLACE.

"Competence" in personal care is described in National Standards, which have been developed in consultation with people working in the care field and approved by employment interests. These standards are used in the assessment by gathering evidence of a candidate's work practice by direct observation or, when this is not possible, by the nearest possible method.

The evidence gathered is then compared to the standards. Candidates are found competent when they consistently fulfil the criteria described in the standards. If a candidate is not able to fulfil the criteria consistently they are judged "not yet competent" and will be helped to develop their practice so that they will be able to show evidence of their competence.

Helpful experience

The assessment system of NVQs/SVQs is intended to be a positive and helpful experience because it focuses attention on what people can do, not what they cannot do yet. Many people find it helpful when finding out about NVQ/SVQ to put aside anything they know about other assessment systems and start from scratch, because this is for most of us an entirely new system.

NVQ/SVQ assessment allows people who have gained their skills, knowledge and understanding by previous education or training, experience in work or in caring for relatives, or as volunteers, to have nationally recognised qualifications. The qualifications themselves are organised so that individuals can build up UNITS as they are able, which add up to a full qualification. Qualifications are awarded at different levels to make progress routes clear and to enable a person to transfer between jobs and work settings more easily.

Discrimination

It is sometimes difficult for care staff to gain education and training. Employers often undervalue the complexity of the tasks in social care and make inadequate provision for teaching new staff or for in-service training. Shift work combined with family responsibilities makes it hard for staff to undertake evening classes. In addition staff have often experienced unfair discrimination in their past education/ schooling, leaving them understandably unwilling to risk further negative experience. There may be discrimination in their present work place which has prevented them from gaining promotion or training. It is vital therefore that the introduction of NVQs/SVQs is not only free from unfair discrimination but that the NVQ assessment system is itself actively anti-racist and anti discriminatory. This means that not only the standards against which the assessment is done are anti-racist and anti discriminatory but that the assessment process and access to the assessment is anti-racist and anti-discriminatory.

The end result of the introduction of NVQs will be that by having better quali-fied and competent staff the quality of care

available to service users will be improved.

It is often assumed that the only way to gain education and training is to go on a course. While this may suit many people it is important to recognise that this is only one way. The over-riding issue is what will work best for you. The separation of training and education and an individual's assessment offered by the NVQ/SVQ system means that how you gain your skills, knowledge and understanding is not part of the way your competence in the work is assessed. This places you in a position where it is up to you to decide how to get the education and training you require. If you are in employment or a volunteer this will obviously be done in conjunction with who ever is in charge of training in your organi-sation and the resources available will affect what is possible. One of the best ways to identify your training, education and assessment needs is to make a plan of what you want, what you need to get what you want, and how you will put it into action.

Your choice

This can then be the basis for you to negotiate your programme of learning. Then within the constraints of the opportunities available you can choose your way or ways to learn. At the same time you should identify your needs for assessment, which can, and I believe should, be a continuous process. In other words, you don't need to wait until you have every-thing settled. Indeed, one way to use the NVQ/SVQ system is to plan to begin assessment on the units you are confident in and progress to units you are not sure of. Then with your assessor's help you can identify areas of work where you need to improve your practice, and discuss what is the best way to do this.

Planning how you will use education, training and assessment is a difficult thing to do on your own. The ideal person to help you would be someone who will encourage you to think things through and express what you want, but will not try to tell you what is best before you have worked it out for yourself. They should also know about the assessment system, so that they can continue to help as you are assessed. They may also be able to help you work out where there is evidence of your competence. Some organisations arrange for a member of staff to fulfil this helping role; they are often called "mentors".

The following five headings may be useful in organising your plan. The questions in each heading are intended to get you thinking: you can ignore them, use them or add to them as you need.

SKILLS NOW

Will the education and training recognise and value the experience, knowledge and understanding that I have already?
I have been doing this work a long time; how can I get recognition for all that experience?

OUTCOME

What changes do I want to make to the way I work?
Do I want to get a different job?
How can I be sure the education and training, once completed, will mean something to employers?

PRACTICAL

Who will pay for it?
Will I get time off to do the education and training?
Do I have to do it all at once or can I do it in parts?
Will I be able to get there?
Is the education and training going to be run at a time suitable to me?

EDUCATIONAL EXPERIENCE

How can I find education and training that is about the real work?

How can I find education and training that I can do?
Will I have to do things I don't like, or know I am not good at?
What will the other people on the education and training be like?
Will I be able to understand?
Will I be able to manage the work?
How will the education and training help me to do the work better?
How will I have a say in the education and training's content?

ANTI-RACISM /ANTI DISCRIMINATION

Will I be discriminated against? You may have this fear because in the past you have been discriminated against. Common examples of discrimination are: because a language other than English is your first language, because you have to leave at a particular time to pick up children, or the building has not been designed for people with disabilities.
Will the education and training help me improve my anti-racist and anti-discriminatory practice?
How can I help to bring about change in the place I work to cater properly for the cultural needs of the people we work with?

ACTION

Work out what is the best way that you learn. Is it:
On your own? With a group of people? Away from work or at work?
Over an extended time, or in short pieces? What works best may depend on what it is you are learning at the time.
When are you able to do this education and training? If you live a busy life, space will have to be made and this space will have to be at a time when you are in the right frame of mind. Education and training is about providing an opportunity for you to learn. For it to be successful it has to be something you can engage with and feel is yours.

Ways to learn

Education and training is offered in a large number of ways, none of which is perfect for all people or all of an individual's needs, so choose what suits you at the time and for the purpose you require. Here are some of the ways you might find useful to learn:

• Learning at work: this may be a pre-planned activity or by planned supervision.
• Short courses: away from your work place or run in the work place for a group of staff.
• Courses in a college: these may be day release, blocks of time, night classes or full-time.
• Open learning: this can be done on your own or with a group of others, using learning materials provided with either tutor support, correspondence or support from other learners. The learning materials used for open learning are also varied - books, work and task sheets, VHF video and interactive video.

Last, and most difficult, you will have to decide how to get what you have decided you want. This may involve some compromise because of what is available. If you are in employment you may find that your employer is only able to offer education and training that is directly linked to the work you do now. This may be fine but it does no harm to ask and to indicate that you may want more in the future. If you are not working in the care field at present, the problems to solve are to locate college or open learning packages that suit you, and to get a grant or another form of financial help.

All about NVQ/SVQs

You can only be assessed for NVQs/SVQs in approved assessment centres. These are places that have proved to the awarding body (the organisations that actually give the NVQ) that they can operate assessment in the proper way. Because NVQs/SVQs are assessed against standards that are work based, approved assessment centres are usually employers or organisations that work with employers who provide assessment. If you cannot gain access to an approved assessment centre you can not be assessed for an NVQ/SVQ, but of course you can prepare yourself to be assessed. The system for operating assessment centres has been in place since September 1990 and it may take some time before there are sufficient assessment centres. If your employer is not part of an assessment centre yet it may be worth enquiring what their plan is. There are costs involved for employers in training staff to be assessors, for example, and for releasing staff to operate the assessment system but it is anticipated that the advantages of the system will outweigh these costs.

All-embracing

NVQ/SVQs in care are part of a much larger system in that will cover all areas of employment. This new system of vocational qualifications is intended to:

• provide qualifications that are valid in the work place
• be easily understood
• enable people to progress
• indicate the level of qualifications so that people can transfer between different types of employment

The focal point of the assessment system is the standards, which are statements of what has to be achieved to do the job well. These standards are agreed by the Care Sector Consortium (representing employment interests) It is important that as you begin to plan your own assessment, you read and become familiar with the standards, which are available in all approved assessment centres. They often appear rather daunting, looking more like telephone books than anything to do with caring for people. Don't let this put you off!

The parts you are likely to use will be reasonably easy to find. Do have a browse through the standards; you may well find units which are about your particular skills which you had not thought of. As the system is developed, more "user friendly" ways of printing the standards are being produced. These will often contain just the units for an award; this is easier to use but do not forget to look at all of the units and awards that are available, since they may suit your needs now or in the future.

Standards are expressed as PERFORMANCE CRITERIA - things that are actually done. These performance criteria are grouped into ELEMENTS, which are in turn grouped into UNITS which describe recognisable pieces of work. Units are grouped together into AWARDS which are set at a level within the NVQ/SVQ framework.

Values in care

The best way in which the "value base" of care can be expressed in the standards, is under review. At present the values are in the CORE PERFORMANCE CRITERIA: candidates have to show evidence that they are fulfilling these core criteria at the same time as they are fulfilling the performance criteria.

This may sound complicated but what it would mean, for example, is that when you are working you are showing respect for your clients (and they are experiencing that respect) as you actually work with them, rather than merely talking about respecting them. The value base of care is clear to most but we are all aware that these values are sometimes absent in the way some individuals and work places operate. The standards have been agreed at a level of best practice, producing minimum requirements of candidates - things they must do to be found competent. The issues to be dealt with in operating assessments

for NVQ/SVQ and the effect on care practice may be seen by looking at one core performance criterion:

The candidate recognises and takes account of the client's culture, political beliefs, race, religion, sexual identity, age, gender, physical and mental condition. *From the Residential, Domiciliary and Day Care Standards.*

The evidence that candidates show of fulfilling the criterion will be different, depending on where and how they work, but to be found competent candidates will have to show that they consistently fulfil the criterion.

It is recognised that in some work places there is racism and discrimination towards the staff and the clients. It will clearly be difficult if not impossible for a candidate to provide sufficient evidence in such work places. This may appear unfair since the racism and/or discrimination may not be the fault of the candidate (indeed they may well be discriminated against themselves). The alternative, of ignoring the candidate's lack of evidence, would be to allow some bad or incomplete practice which would devalue the awards and not contribute to the development of improved practice. Therefore in such circumstances the assessment for NVQ/SVQ will have assisted in identifying an important task for the work place - removing the discrimination or racism. This is a task primarily related to the requirements of justice, good care practise and the law. NVQs/SVQs can not in themselves achieve such improvements, but because the standards are based on good practice, assessors do work within organisations that are taking action to improve practice, anti-racism and anti-discrimination.

The assessment process

The basics of the assessment process are:
• Evidence is gathered of the candidate's

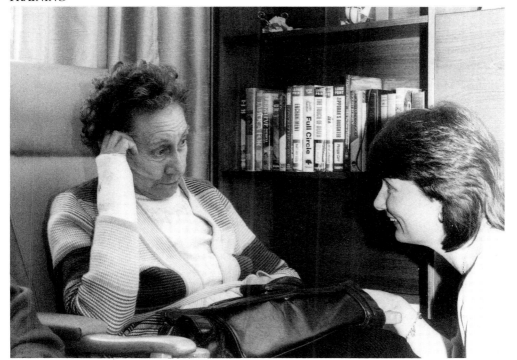

The "value base" of care means that you are showing respect for your clients as you work with them.

competence in conditions as close as possible to the conditions under which they would normally work.

• The assessor must ensure that the candidate is consistently fulfilling all the performance criteria of the unit(s) on which they are being assessed, before they can be found competent.

• If a candidate does not show sufficient evidence for one or more performance criteria in a unit, then they are not yet competent in that unit.

Filling the gaps

Assessment is not therefore a one-off examination. There will be many people who on the initial gathering of evidence will have evidence gaps. Such gaps are of three types:

1. There is some difficulty in gathering the evidence which will have to be overcome. (Assessors are prepared for their task and to find other ways of gathering evidence.)

2. The timetable to gather sufficient evidence has been under-estimated and the candidate and the assessor will have to plan again.

3. The candidate is not performing up to the standard required and therefore needs to improve their practice. (It is important to recognise that one reason for this may well be that the policy and practice of the work place itself is at fault.)

The only way for the assessment process to start is for the candidate to request assessment. Once the assessor has been assigned to the candidate they need to plan the assessment. They must ensure that they are both clear about the basis they will work on. Before the candidate and the assessor can begin the actual assessment process a number of questions have to be talked through and agreed by both the candidate and the assessor:

• What are the units of competence the candidate wants to be assessed?

• How is the candidate going to provide the assessor with evidence of their competence?

• What evidence gathering methods will be appropriate, for example how will the rights and privacy of clients be ensured?

• What is the type and range of evidence that will need to be shown for the assessor to be satisfied that the candidate consistently fulfils the criteria?

• How will the evidence be recorded, and who will have access to those records?

• Can the records be used for anything other than the assessment?

• How will the assessor ensure that the evidence gathering methods used will not unfairly discriminate against the candidate?

• How will the candidate be given feedback on their performance?

• When will the evidence gathering start and the assessment made on the evidence be finished?

• What is the appeals procedure?

• What are the education and training opportunities - especially if there are areas where the candidate is found not yet competent?

Competence

Once agreed, the evidence gathering can begin. This is primarily the candidate bringing to the attention of the assessor actual evidence and/or parts of their work that they believe will show evidence of their competence. This evidence may well be about work that the candidate has done before and records in some way their achievement. This is one of the times when the candidate will be glad that they have spent time planning for the assessment. As more people use the NVQ/SVQ system there will develop a better understanding of how best to use it. Therefore do seek out others who are going through assessment; you can offer each other support.

As the candidate is found competent in the units they have asked to be assessed on they will receive a certificate for each unit. When they have been found competent for all the units in an award they will get a certificate which will give the name of the award and its level. Awards at the same NVQ/SVQ level in the care sector, even if from different awarding bodies, are recognised as being equivalent. You are advised to keep these certificates (and any others you have) safe. The National Record of Vocational Achievement(NROVA) is a grey plastic box file designed to keep certificates and records together.

Your future

The NVQ/SVQ system is designed to encourage people to build up their qualifications, either to progress in their present work or to transfer into other areas of work. When you have achieved your first award, consider how you would like to progress. Such progression may be into other areas of competence at the same level or into higher levels including full professional qualification. For example level 3 NVQ/SVQ Awards in Care are recognised as part of an entry to the Diploma in Social Work.

The work that has gone into the development of National Vocational Qualifications, Scottish Vocational Qualifications and associated education and training has been undertaken by a large number of individuals and groups. One of the major strengths of these developments is that they are based on collective work which draws upon the perspectives of all involved and associated with care work. In this chapter I have attempted to represent this collective work in a concise manner, but the work remains that of the original authors and working groups.

Views and opinions expressed are mine and not necessarily those of the Central Council for Education and Training in Social Work.

CHAPTER 18

Useful addresses

Resources you can draw on for practical help, information and publications

All these organisations welcome a stamped, self-addressed envelope sent with your enquiry.

Action for Dysphasic Adults, Canterbury House, 1 Royal Street, London SE1 7LN. Tel: 071 261 9572. Advice and information for people with speech difficulties, their families and carers.

Age Concern England, Astral House, 1268 London Road, London SW16 4ER. Tel: 081 679 8000. Information and publications. Practical volunteer services through local groups.

Age Exchange Reminiscence Centre, 11 Blackheath Village, London SE3 9LA. Tel: 081 318 9105. A unique reminiscence centre and hands-on museum. Activities include reminiscence groups, youth theatre, professional touring reminiscence theatre company, book publication, exhibitions and a comprehensive programme of reminiscence training courses such as "Introduction to reminiscence", "Making shows, books and exhibitions", "Reminiscence with mentally infirm elderly people", and "Cross-generational reminiscence".

Alzheimer's Disease Society, 158-160 Balham High Road, London SW12 9BN. Tel: 081 675 6557/8/9/0. National Association and local branches providing carers with information and support; newsletter and other publications.

Arthritis Care, 5 Grosvenor Crescent, London SW1X 7ER. Tel: 071 235 0902. Self-help support group (local branches) for arthritis sufferers.

Association of Continence Advisers, at the Disabled Living Foundation, 380-384 Harrow Road, London W9 2HU. Tel: 071 289 6111. Network of professional nurse continence advisers.

British Association of the Hard of Hearing, 7-11 Armstrong Road, London W3 7JL. Tel: 081 743 1110. Runs local clubs in many parts of the country; also provides information and a newsletter.

British Colostomy Association, 38-39 Eccleston Square, London SW1V 1PB. Tel: 071 828 5175. Officers and volunteers give personal advice and help to those with colostomies.

British Deaf Association, 38 Victoria Place, Carlisle. Tel: 0228 48844. Information, services and clubs for people born deaf and using sign language.

British Diabetic Association, 10 Queen Anne Street, London W1M 0BD. 071 323 1531. Information, publications and services for diabetic people and their carers.

British Epilepsy Association, Anstey House, 40 Hanover Square, Leeds LS3 1BE. Tel: 0532 439393. Advice, information, self-help groups.

British Red Cross Society, 9 Grosvenor Crescent, London SW1X 7EJ. Tel: 071 235 5454. Volunteer beauty care and other services.

Centre for Policy on Ageing, 25-31 Ironmonger Row, London EC1V 3QP. Tel: 071 253 1787. Publications and information on old age, policy and service provision, including practical handbooks on aspects of residential care. Publishes Home Life: a code of practice for residential care, the guidance document for the Registered Homes Act 1984.

Christian Council on Ageing, The Old Court, Greens Norton, Nr Towcester, Northants NN12 8BS. Tel: 0327 50481. Information and publications on spiritual needs in old age; local branches.

Counsel and Care for the Elderly, Twyman House, 16 Bonny Street, London NW1 9PG. Tel: 071 485 1550. Assists elderly people into residential and nursing homes. Advice and casework counselling service.

Cruse-Bereavement Care, Cruse House, 126 Sheen Road, Richmond, Surrey TW9 1UR. Tel: 081 940 4818. Service of counselling, advice and opportunities for social contact for all bereaved people.

Disabled Living Foundation, 380-384 Harrow Road, London W9 2HU. Tel: 071 289 6111. Publications and information, especially on incontinence, clothing, aids and equipment, music, visual handicap and footwear.

Gardens for the Disabled Trust and Garden Club, Mrs Julia Sebline, Hayes Farmhouse, Hayes Lane, Peasmarsh, E. Sussex. Tel: 0424 882345. Practical and financial assistance for disabled people wanting to take an active part in gardening.

Help the Aged, 16-18 St James's Walk, Clerkenwell, London EC1R 0BE. Tel: 071 253 0253. Publications and information. Specialist services include skilled reminiscence work with confused elderly people.

Horticultural Therapy, Goulds Ground, Vallis Way, Frome, Somerset BA11 3DW. Tel: 0373 64782. Technical, advisory and support service to gardening projects.

MIND/National Association for Mental Health. 22 Harley Street, London W1N 2ED. Aims to promote mental health and help mentally disordered people. Local associations throughout the country.

Multiple Sclerosis Society of Great Britain and Northern Ireland, 25 Effie Road, Fulham, London SW6 1EE. Tel: 071 736 6267.

National Deaf Blind League, 18 Rainbow Court, Paston Ridings, Peterborough PE4 6UP. Tel: 0733 73511. Information, advice and publications, including illustrated instructions for manual alphabets.

National Schizophrenia Fellowship, 28 Castle Street, Kingston-upon-Thames, Surrey KT1 1SS. Tel:081 547 3937. Advisory service through the national office. 120 local groups.

Nottingham Rehab Ltd, 17 Ludlow Hill Road, Melton Road, West Bridgford, Nottingham NG2 6HD. Tel: 0602 452345. A variety of activity materials and aids – catalogue available.

Nutrition Advisory Group for the Elderly (British Dietetic Association). Information and a handbook,

Eating through the '90s, for those providing meals for elderly people. Available from Elizabeth Haughton, Dept. Nutrition and Dietetics, Gloucestershire Royal Hospital, Great Western Road, Gloucester GL1 3NN.

Orientation Aids, Dalebank, Glencaple, Dumfries. Books and reality orientation materials.

Royal National Institute for the Blind, 224 Great Portland Street, London W1N 6AA. Tel: 071 388 1266. Advice, information and publications, especially Braille books, periodicals and music, and Moon books and periodicals.

Royal National Institute for the Deaf, 105 Gower Street, London WC1E 6AH. Tel: 071 387 8033. Advice, information and services to people with impaired hearing those working with them.

Schizophrenia Association of Great Britain. Bryn Hyfryd, The Crescent, Bangor, Gwynedd LL57 2AG. Tel: 0248 354048. A telephone and postal advice service is offered to psychiatric patients, their relatives and mental health professionals.

Social Service Departments – at your local authority. The address will be in the telephone directory, or available from your local library. Residential home registration officers are a source of information and advice; specialist social workers can help with handicaps such as deafness or blindness.

Talking Books for the Handicapped (National Listening Library), 12 Lant Street, London SE1 1QR. Tel: 071 407 9417. A postal lending library service of literature recorded on long-playing cassettes.

TFH, 76 Barracks Road, Sandy Lane Industrial Estate, Stourport-on-Severn, Worcestershire DY13 9QB. Tel: 0299 827820. Games, puzzles, pastimes etc for older people.

University of the Third Age, 1 Stockwell Green, SW9 9JF. Tel: 071 737 2541. Promotes and organises self-help educational activities for older people.

Winslow Press, Telford Road, Bicester, Oxfordshire OX6 0TS. Tel: 0869 244733. Books, especially on aspects of caring for the elderly mentally infirm, activity aids and games, reminiscence materials.

Glossary of terms

Abdomen. The stomach or belly. This area of the body is described as extending from just under the rib cage down to the top of the thighs.

Affect (see also Mood). The emotional state or "mood" of a person.

AIDS (**Acquired Immunodeficiency Syndrome** - see also HIV). AIDS is a condition caused by a virus called HIV (Human Immunodeficiency Virus). This damages the body's defence system so that it cannot fight infection. AIDS causes many people to develop certain forms of cancer, and to get serious infections of the lungs, digestive system, the brain and skin. It is passed on by exchanging body fluids such as blood, semen and vaginal fluids.

Alzheimer's disease (see also Dementia). A form of dementia characterised by changes to the brain, although the particular cause is unknown. Disorientation, loss of memory, loss of intellectual function, apathy as well as difficulty with coordinating movement, speech or thoughts, are common features.

Amnesia. Loss of memory.

Analgesics. Medicines that provide relief from pain. The commonest and most simple analgesics include aspirin and paracetamol. Stronger types of analgesia may be addictive, for example morphine.

Angina. A tight strangling sensation of chest pain, usually on exertion. This is due to narrowing or blockage of the arteries that supply blood to the heart muscle, resulting in insufficient blood supply.

Anorexia. The loss of desire to eat. Emotional disturbances such as depression may induce a chronic state of anorexia.

Antidepressant drugs. Medicines that are used in the treatment of depression. These drugs act upon and stimulate parts of the nervous system. Some functions of the nervous system may be reduced with normal ageing.

Anus (see also Colon). The muscular ring at the end of the intestinal canal. The end of the pelvic colon.

Anxiety state. A condition in which the individual is so worried about a certain situation or problem, that their life is severely restricted. The main characteristic is the inability to relax.

Arteriosclerosis. A gradual loss of elasticity in the walls of arteries, due to thickening and the build up of calcium deposits. There is decreased blood flow and oxygen supply to essential parts of the brain and body. It is one of the causes of dementia.

Arthritis (see also Osteoarthritis and Rheumatoid arthritis). Inflammation causing pain, stiffness and swelling in one or more joints. There may be serious deformity (eg of the hands) and disability. There are several different types of arthritis, including osteoarthritis and rheumatoid arthritis. Main causes are inflammation, and the effects of wear and tear.

Behaviour modification. A programme in which a specific goal or reward is provided to correct an inappropriate behaviour. It is repeatedly reinforced over a period of days or weeks. Screaming or shouting may be lessened, for example, by providing regular individual attention when the person is not shouting or screaming.

Blood pressure (see also Hypertension). The force of blood in the arteries measured in millimetres of mercury by a machine called a sphygmomanometer. Blood pressures are written down as two figures. The top figure is called the "systolic" and the bottom figure is known as the "diastolic". How high or low blood pressure is depends on the strength of the heart beat and the condition of the arteries.

Burn-out (see also Stress). A reaction to stress which may take various forms. The individual becomes unable to cope with all the physical and emotional demands made upon them.

Chronic. A term used to describe a long-standing

and continuing disease process marked by progressive deterioration (sometimes despite treatment).

Cognition. Consciously knowing, understanding and having insight into personal and environmental events. The person may not necessarily be able to take action.

Colon (see also Anus). A part of the large intestine that absorbs nutrients and fluid from the diet. It ends at the anus.

Concussion. Brief loss of consciousness produced by a knock to the head. The person becomes very pale, has a feeble pulse and shallow breathing.

Confusional states. Conditions in which consciousness is clouded, so that the individual is unable to think clearly or act rationally. Confusional states may be temporary, due to acute illness (toxic confusional states), or long term and irreversible.

Connective tissue. The supporting tissues of the body, found under the skin, between muscles, and supporting blood vessels and nerves. Their functions are mainly mechanical, connecting other active tissues and organs.

Constipation. Incomplete or infrequent action of the bowels, due to lack of muscle activity, insufficient fluids or inadequate diet.

Continence (see also Incontinence). The ability to control the functions of passing urine or faeces when desired.

Compulsive disorder. An impulse to carry out or repeat certain actions. They may be recognised as being meaningless, but the person cannot stop carrying out these actions. The compulsion becomes so great that the person is unable to carry out their normal daily activities.

Cramp. Painful contraction of a muscle, associated with salt loss through lack of fluids, or reaction to poisons of various kinds, affecting a muscle or the nerves controlling it.

CVA (Cerebrovascular accident). See Stroke.

Dehydration. Excessive loss of fluid from the body caused by vomiting, diarrhoea or sweating, or from the lack of adequate fluid intake.

Delirium tremens (see also Withdrawal). This occurs when people highly dependent upon alcohol or drugs are suddenly deprived of them. The person may become very irritable or confused, and suffer delusions or hallucinations. Physical signs may include sweating, a rapid pulse and sleeplessness.

Delusion. An irrational belief or attitude that is out of keeping with a person's background. Delusions cannot be corrected by appeals to reason. The ideas are not shared by anyone else.

Dementia (see also Alzheimer's disease). An organic mental illness caused by changes to the brain. This may be a result of disease or damage. The principal changes include inability to learn and retain information, inability to recall recent events, and feelings of anxiety and depression. This leads to disorientation and confused behaviour.

Depression. The commonest functional condition encountered in older people. It is a morbid sadness which is distinct from that which normally accompanies bereavement or loss. Its features include reduced enjoyment, slowness and a lack of interest in life or the lives of others.

Diabetes. Failure of the pancreas in the body to produce insulin, or failure of the body to use the insulin sufficiently. Insulin breaks down sugary foods, allowing the body to use them for energy. Diabetes results in too much sugar circulating in the blood. Normal body functioning, for example wound healing, is affected by the condition.

Disorientation. A state of confusion in which an individual has lost a sense of where they are, what time it is and what they are doing.

Dysarthria. Difficulty in producing speech, due to disruption of the nerve supply to the muscles needed. Understanding of language is not affected, nor the ability to decide what to say.

Dysphasia. Disturbance of the ability to produce or understand language, which may affect understanding, speech, reading and writing.

Epilepsy. A condition in which excessive or disorganised electrical activity in the brain causes fits. These may involve the whole body with loss of consciousness (*grand mal*) or parts of the body, with perhaps a short loss of full consciousness, known as *petit mal* fits. "Focal fits" are said to occur when only one part of the body is affected.

Exertion. The amount of effort, physical or mental, a person puts into carrying out a task.

Faeces. Waste matter that is indigestible such as cellulose food (fibre), excreted by the bowel.

Fainting. A temporary loss of consciousness due to a fall in blood pressure. The person usually falls to the floor, as this is the way in which the body attempts to help the blood circulation, so that more oxygen can reach the brain.

Fracture. A broken bone. The signs and symptoms include pain, swelling, loss of power and shortening of the affected limb. A fracture at the point where the thigh bone is connected to the hip usually results in the limb being turned to the side.

Fibre (in diet). The term is used to describe food that is high in roughage, indigestible, which stimulates the action of the intestine.

Functional. Functional mental disorders are those for which no definite physical cause has yet been found. They cover a wide spectrum, from mild degrees of anxiety and depression to serious illnesses where the person is unable to cope with life. They may have severe symptoms such as hallucinations and delusions.

Genital. Relating to the sexual organs of the man or woman.

Guarding. A defensive action that a person may take to safeguard themselves or to prevent any pain. It may include not wishing to talk about difficult subjects or holding oneself in a comfortable position that prevents physical pain.

Hallucinations. A false perception that a person can see, hear, smell, taste and touch something that exists only to themselves and not to other people.

HIV (Human Immunodeficiency Virus). The virus that causes AIDS. It is not one virus, but a family of many similar viruses. It weakens the body's defence system by entering and destroying white cells that normally protect the body from infection.

Huntington's chorea. A chronic disease that is passed on through family heredity. The mental and physical powers of the person are affected, leading to a type of dementia. It is usually characterised by profound stiffness, rigidity, and difficulty with speech and swallowing.

Hypertension (see also Blood Pressure). A condition in which the blood pressure is higher than it should be.

Hypomania (see also Mania and Mood). Used to describe a degree of elation, excitement and activity that is higher than normal. It is considered to be less severe than mania.

Hypothermia. Body temperature below the usual value of 37 degrees centigrade. At about 35 degrees centigrade confusion and listlessness may begin. Below 33 degrees centigrade the breathing and pulse rate and blood pressure may start to fall. If prolonged, death may occur.

Incontinence (see also Continence). The inability to control the passage of urine or faeces until a suitable time and place is found. Urinary incontinence may occur when abdominal pressure, eg through coughing or lifting heavy weights, causes urine to leak from the bladder and urethra. Faecal incontinence is caused by a loss of control of the anus. Disorientation may also cause incontinence.

Insomnia. Difficulty getting to sleep or remaining asleep for long.

Intoxication (see also Toxin). Poisoning by drugs or harmful substances. This may also include a state of drunkenness produced by too much alcohol.

Intractable. Used to describe any condition that is difficult to control or cure.

Larynx. The organ of the voice. Across it are spread the vocal cords of elastic tissue, and the vibrations and contractions of these produce the changes in the pitch of the voice.

Mania (see also Hypomania and Mood). Elevated mood and extreme excitement, accompanied by acceleration of both thoughts and actions.

Medication (see also Sedation and Tranquilliser). Used to describe tablets, liquids or injections that are used to improve a person's physical or mental condition.

Meningitis. A serious infection of the tissues surrounding the brain.

Metabolism. The process of life. The need, for example, to eat, drink and sleep, and for the body to use the food and fluids to continue to work and repair tissue damage when required.

Mood (see also Hypomania and Mania). The mood of a person, feeling happy or sad, can be affected by many factors. Also known as the "affect", the main features are elation or depression, with anxiety and agitation.

Motor strength. Strength that permits action of the limbs and body to move about. This usually includes the muscle and connective tissue that make up the series of levers and pulleys within the body.

Neurosis. Neuroses are common conditions whose symptoms include anxiety, phobias, compulsive states and hysterical reactions. The person's personality and understanding of their problem usually remain intact, although they are still often unable to help themselves.

Organic. Relating to a body organ. The term is used to describe a disease process that has a known physical cause. Dementia for example is a result of damage to the brain.

Osteoarthritis (see also Arthritis). A form of arthritis. It usually affects older people and larger joints. The cause is unknown but sufferers may be prone to more wear and tear of joints. There is destruction of the spongy pads (cartilage) between the bones, and formation of small bony outgrowths at the edges of the bone joint.

Paralysis. Loss of movement (but not necessarily sensation) in a muscle or group of muscles normally under the person's control. May be due to damage to the muscle itself or to its nerve supply.

Paraphrenia. Schizophrenia occurring for the first time in later life. The person usually retains their personality, but may experience delusions and hallucinations. They may be very suspicious, and unable to think clearly or act rationally. It can be made worse by the inability to see or hear properly.

Parkinsonism. Symptoms that are similar to Parkinson's disease: shaking or trembling, rhythmical muscular tremors, rigidity and a mask-like face that shows no emotion. Thumb and fore fingers may move in a "rolling" fashion. It can be caused by tranquillisers used to treat mental health problems.

Personality disorder. Used to describe conditions where a person's lifelong characteristics cause suffering either to themselves or to society. The concept is controversial, and has been used to describe people who are "inadequate", or who are constantly very suspicious of individuals and society. This may make them act in a way that is unacceptable to others.

Phobia. An irrational fear which is so strong that it interferes with day-to-day life.

Prognosis. The outlook for a person with a disease, in terms of death and disability.

Psychosocial. Relating to factors that are both social and psychological in origin; the relationship between one-to-one and group interaction.

Psychosis. Severe mental illness where the symptoms affect the whole person. They often lose touch with reality, have no insight into their condition, and act in a way which does not fit into acceptable patterns of life. The person's personality may be affected by delusions and hallucinations.

Reality orientation. The way in which older people with mental illness are helped to keep in touch with the world around them. This may be through the individual use of large clocks, signs on doors and newspapers. It can also be used in groups where older people are encouraged to participate in activities that remind them, for example, of where they are and the time of year.

Reclusiveness. The characteristics of a person who wishes to remain alone, isolated, not wanting to join in or be involved with other people.

Recovery position. The safest position in which to

place a person who is unconscious or concussed. The purpose is to ensure that their mouth is kept open to allow them to breath and to ensure that saliva, vomit or blood can flow out rather than going into the lungs. Movement should be minimal, rolling the person onto their left side where possible. If a back injury is suspected, this should only be done as a life-saving measure.

Rehabilitation. The process by which health workers restore a person who has had a serious illness to as near as possible their state of health before the illness.

Reminiscence therapy. This may involve active participation by individuals or groups, using past life events to understand the reasons for their mental health problems. Or it can be an activity session, using objects and photographs from the past to stimulate discussion, and reinforce an individual's sense of personal identity. The past can also be used as a basis to share concerns and anxieties, since people with dementia are more likely to have a better memory for events long ago than for more recent events.

Rheumatoid arthritis (see also Arthritis). A form of arthritis occurring in the small and large joints. It is usually characterised by chronic inflammation. Little is known about the cause.

Rheumatism. Term loosely applied in ordinary speech to any pain of unknown cause in the joints or muscles.

Sedative (see also Medication and Tranquilliser). A drug which reduces excitement, anxiety and tension.

Senile dementia (see Dementia). Dementia occurring in old age.

Shock. This may arise out of fear or pain; it may also be the result of loss of blood, or a reaction to medicines, or electrical currents. There is a sudden fall in blood pressure, which if untreated will lead to a lack of oxygen in the tissues.

Sprain. An injury to a ligament when the joint it is supporting is forced through a range of movements greater than normal, without dislocation or fracture.

Stroke. A brain disorder of rapid onset, usually caused by a blockage in or haemorrhage (bleeding) from one of the main arteries of the brain. Speech and movement are most commonly affected but other functions may be damaged, depending upon which part of the brain is involved. The speed of recovery depends on the extent of the blockage or haemorrhage. Also known as a cerebrovascular accident (CVA).

Syphilis. A contagious disease passed on by sexual activity. The early infectious stage may be followed by a latent period of many years when serious nerve and vascular problems arise. This late consequence of untreated syphilis (General Paralysis of the Insane) is less common since the improvement of routine screening and early treatment.

Stress (see also Burn-out). The reaction, both physical and mental, to the demands made upon a person. Stress reactions occur when the individual is unable to cope with all the demands made upon them.

Therapeutic. Relating to the science and art of treating people. Therapy may be in the form of medical or surgical treatment, but also involves personal approaches, such as listening, counselling or providing the right environment in which a person feels comfortable and safe.

Thought disorder. This describes the abnormal speed or content of thoughts or the mixed up way that thoughts may occur to a person. There may be thought withdrawal (thoughts coming to an abrupt end), and thought insertion (extra thoughts that do not relate to the current situation).

Toxin. Any poisonous compound. Toxins may be released by bacteria multiplying in the body in an infection.

Tranquilliser (see also Medication and Sedation). Medicines that allay anxiety and have a calming effect on the person. They may also prevent them from feeling pain.

Trauma. A wound or injury. Emotional trauma such as bereavement can give rise to mental illness.

Tumour. A lump or swelling in the body that is not inflamed. A "benign" tumour does not infiltrate or grow in other parts of the body. A "malignant" tumour may spread into other organs.

Urethra. The tube that carries urine from the bladder to outside the body.

Urinary tract infection. An infection that affects the bladder or the urethra. It usually results in the person wanting to pass urine frequently, sometimes causing pain and a stinging sensation when this happens.

Vascular. Relating to blood vessels, usually arteries or veins.

Varicose veins. A condition, usually of the lower leg, in which the veins are swollen and may be twisted due to structural changes in the walls or valves of the vessels. These veins have difficulty returning blood back to the heart. Knocks to varicose veins commonly cause leg ulcers in older people.

Vertigo. A feeling of dizziness accompanied by a feeling that either oneself or one's surroundings are spinning.

Withdrawal (from drugs, alcohol - see also Delerium tremens). The physical and mental symptoms experienced by a person when stopping alcohol or drugs that their body has come to depend upon.

Index